Tracheobronchial, Pulmonary and Mediastinal Problems in General Thoracic Surgery

Guest Editor

STEVEN R. DEMEESTER, MD

SURGICAL CLINICS
OF NORTH AMERICA

www.surgical.theclinics.com

Consulting Editor
RONALD F. MARTIN, MD

October 2010 • Volume 90 • Number 5

SAUNDERS an imprint of ELSEVIER, Inc.

W.B. SAUNDERS COMPANY

A Division of Elsevier Inc.

1600 John F. Kennedy Blvd., Suite 1800, Philadelphia, PA 19103-2899

http://www.theclinics.com

SURGICAL CLINICS OF NORTH AMERICA Volume 90, Number 5

October 2010 ISSN 0039–6109, ISBN-13: 978-1-4377-2615-2

Editor: John Vassallo, j.vassallo@elsevier.com

Developmental Editor: Donald Mumford

Surgical Clinics of North America (ISSN 0039–6109) is published bimonthly by Elsevier Inc., 360 Park Avenue South, New York, NY 10010-1710. Months of publication are February, April, June, August, October, and December. Business and Editorial Offices: 1600 John F. Kennedy Blvd., Suite 1800, Philadelphia, PA 19103-2899. Periodicals postage paid at New York, NY and additional mailing offices. Subscription prices are $291.00 per year for US individuals, $475.00 per year for US institutions, $145.00 per year for US students and residents, $356.00 per year for Canadian individuals, $590.00 per year for Canadian institutions, $401.00 for international individuals, $590.00 per year for international institutions and $200.00 per year for Canadian and foreign students/residents. To receive student/resident rate, orders must be accompanied by name of affiliated institution, date of term, and the *signature* of program/residency coordinator on institution letterhead. Orders will be billed at individual rate until proof of status is received. Foreign air speed delivery is included in all *Clinics* subscription prices. All prices are subject to change without notice. POSTMASTER: Send address changes to *Surgical Clinics*, Elsevier Health Sciences Division, Subscription Customer Service, 3251 Riverport Lane, Maryland Heights, MO 63043. **Customer Service (orders, claims, online, change of address): Telephone: 1-800-654-2452 (U.S. and Canada); 314-447-8871 (outside U.S. and Canada). Fax: 314-447-8029. E-mail: journalscustomerservice-usa@elsevier.com (for print support); journalsonline support-usa@elsevier.com (for online support).**

Reprints. For copies of 100 or more, of articles in this publication, please contact the Commercial Reprints Department, Elsevier Inc., 360 Park Avenue South, New York, New York 10010-1710. Tel. (212) 633-3812, Fax: (212) 462-1935, e-mail: reprints@elsevier.com.

The Surgical Clinics of North America is also published in Spanish by McGraw-Hill Interamericana Editores S.A., P.O. Box 5-237 06500 Mexico D.F. Mexico; and in Portuguese by Interlivros Edicoes Ltda., Rua Comandante Coelho 1085, CEP 21250, Rio de Janeiro, Brazil; and in Greek by Paschalidis Medical Publications, Athens Greece.

The Surgical Clinics of North America is covered in *MEDLINE/PubMed (Index Medicus)*, *EMBASE/Excerpta Medica*, *Current Contents/Clinical Medicine*, *Current Contents/Life Sciences*, *Science Citation Index*, and *ISI/BIOMED*.

Printed and bound by CPI Group (UK) Ltd, Croydon, CR0 4YY

Transferred to Digital Print 2011

Contributors

CONSULTING EDITOR

RONALD F. MARTIN, MD
Staff Surgeon, Department of Surgery, Marshfield Clinic, Marshfield, Wisconsin; Clinical Associate Professor, University of Wisconsin School of Medicine and Public Health, Madison, Wisconsin; Colonel, Medical Corps, United States Army Reserve

GUEST EDITOR

STEVEN R. DEMEESTER, MD
Associate Professor of Cardiothoracic Surgery, University of Southern California, Keck School of Medicine, Los Angeles, California

AUTHORS

CARL L. BACKER, MD
A.C. Buehler Professor of Surgery, Division of Cardiovascular-Thoracic Surgery, Children's Memorial Hospital; Professor of Surgery, Northwestern University Feinberg School of Medicine, Chicago, Illinois

FARZANEH BANKI, MD
Assistant Professor, Department of Cardiothoracic and Vascular Surgery, The University of Texas Medical School at Houston, Houston, Texas

ROSS BREMNER, MD, PhD
Chief, Thoracic Surgery, Surgical Director, Center for Thoracic Disease, The Heart and Lung Institute, St Joseph's Hospital and Medical Center, Phoenix, Arizona

JAMES BURNS, MD
Assistant in Surgery, Division of Thoracic and Laryngeal Surgery, Massachusetts General Hospital; Assistant Professor of Surgery, Harvard Medical School, Boston, Massachusetts

NEIL A. CHRISTIE, MD
Assistant Professor of Surgery, Department of Cardiothoracic Surgery, University of Pittsburgh Medical Center, Pittsburgh, Pennsylvania

HIRAN C. FERNANDO, MBBS, FRCS
Department of Cardiothoracic Surgery, Boston Medical Center, Boston University School of Medicine, Boston, Massachusetts

HENNING A. GAISSERT, MD
Associate Visiting Surgeon, Division of Thoracic and Laryngeal Surgery, Massachusetts General Hospital; Associate Professor of Surgery, Department of Surgery, Harvard Medical School, Boston, Massachusetts

WAYNE L. HOFSTETTER, MD
Associate Professor, Department of Thoracic and Cardiovascular Surgery, The University of Texas MD Anderson, Houston, Texas

SEEMA KAPUR, MD
Division of Thoracic Surgery, Swedish Cancer Institute and Medical Center, Seattle, Washington

JAE Y. KIM, MD
Thoracic Surgery Fellow, Department of Thoracic and Cardiovascular Surgery, The University of Texas MD Anderson Cancer Center, Houston, Texas

ELBERT KUO, MD, MPH
Heart and Lung Institute, St Joseph's Hospital and Medical Center, Phoenix, Arizona

BRIAN E. LOUIE, MD, FRCSC, FACS
Division of Thoracic Surgery, Swedish Cancer Institute and Medical Center, Seattle, Washington

MARY S. MAISH, MD, MPH
Associate Clinical Professor of Surgery, University of California Los Angeles David Geffen School of Medicine, Los Angeles, California

BRYAN F. MEYERS, MD, MPH
Professor of Surgery, Division of Cardiothoracic Surgery, Department of Surgery, Washington University School of Medicine, Saint Louis, Missouri

DANIEL P. RAYMOND, MD
Assistant Professor of Surgery, Division of Thoracic and Foregut Surgery, Department of Surgery, University of Rochester School of Medicine and Dentistry, Rochester, New York

HYDE M. RUSSELL, MD
Assistant Professor of Surgery, Division of Cardiovascular-Thoracic Surgery, Children's Memorial Hospital, Chicago, Illinois

NICHOLAS R. THIESSEN, MD
Surgical Resident, St Joseph's Hospital and Medical Center, Phoenix, Arizona

VICTOR VAN BERKEL, MD, PhD
Associate Professor of Surgery, Division of Cardiothoracic Surgery, Department of Surgery, University of Louisville School of Medicine, Louisville, Kentucky

THOMAS J. WATSON, MD, FACS
Associate Professor of Surgery, Chief of Thoracic Surgery, Division of Thoracic and Foregut Surgery, Department of Surgery, University of Rochester School of Medicine and Dentistry, Rochester, New York

YIFAN ZHENG, BS
Department of Cardiothoracic Surgery, Boston Medical Center, Boston University School of Medicine, Boston, Massachusetts

Contents

procedures. Despite advances in anesthesia, including the use of epidural analgesics, and advances in surgical techniques and perioperative care, postoperative pulmonary complications remain the leading cause of morbidity and mortality in thoracic surgery. No single parameter is predictive of postoperative complications or mortality in patients who undergo a thoracic procedure. Therefore, patients should not be denied for surgical resection based on any single abnormal test or parameter. A comprehensive assessment of the functional status, exercise tolerance, and pulmonary function should be performed before surgery to select the patients appropriately, predict the risk of postoperative complications, and achieve better outcomes.

Hemoptysis and thoracic fungal infections are infrequent but challenging problems, especially when encountered in the emergency setting. The evaluation and management of massive and nonmassive hemoptysis is described with special attention to radiologic, bronchcoscopic, and surgical interventions. The important principles of airway control, stabilization, and definitive management are emphasized. Endemic and opportunistic fungal infections are more common than they seem. The role of the surgeon is to assist in diagnosis, evaluate and treat pulmonary nodules, and consider resectional therapy for mycetoma and invasive fungal infections in selected candidates.

The solitary pulmonary nodule is a common finding on radiographic studies performed for other reasons. It is important that the probability of malignancy be assessed when these nodules are found. This chapter outlines a diagnostic approach for these nodules to optimize non-invasive and invasive testing, and describes the value of the various modalities used to evaluate these abnormalities.

Primary tumors of the mediastinum and chest wall comprise a diverse group of conditions with a wide range of presentations. A thorough knowledge of thoracic anatomy is essential for appropriate diagnosis and treatment. Given their proximity to critical structures, treatment of these tumors is often challenging. Although surgery is the mainstay of therapy for most mediastinal and chest wall tumors, a multidisciplinary approach is valuable in many cases.

Resection of pulmonary metastases is reasonable and is commonly performed for patients whose primary disease is controlled and for whom the metastatic burden in the chest is such that all disease can be resected safely. The use of video- assisted thoracic surgery rather than an open approach in metastasectomy, however, is still being debated. In addition, nonresectional therapies such as radiofrequency ablation and stereotactic body radiation therapy are being used in centers for patients with oligometastases to the lungs. This article reviews the indications and approaches for surgical resection, as well as these other nonresectional therapies. At present, it is difficult to directly compare these approaches because of the heterogeneous nature of metastasectomy series. Moreover, the stereotactic body radiation therapy and radiofrequency ablation studies have involved smaller numbers of patients and shorter follow-up than the surgical studies. The preliminary data for these nonresectional therapies, however, are encouraging and certainly should be considered in the decision tree when treating patients with pulmonary metastases.

THE CLINICS ARE NOW AVAILABLE ONLINE!

Access your subscription at:
www.theclinics.com

Foreword

Tracheobronchial, Pulmonary, and Mediastinal Problems in General Thoracic Surgery

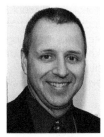

Ronald F. Martin, MD
Consulting Editor

We all tend to see the world through a prism of our own creation. I am no different. As I write this Foreword, I find myself preoccupied with thoughts of returning to war. I don't share this with the readership because my personal activities are of any consequence but, rather, that I am struck by how it changes my opinion about what I feel is necessary to know.

One of the great tensions in the discipline of general surgery at this time is how "general" should a general surgeon be or how specialized or focused should he or she be? There appears to be a great deal of ambivalence on this topic. Patients like to deal with one person with whom they can develop a relationship and trust but they also want their surgeons to be extremely practiced at whatever problem they need solved. Our certifying authorities want to maintain a depth and breadth of superior knowledge and competency in many areas but our educational regulatory agencies want us to limit residents' work hours and subsequently their exposure to opportunities to learn. Many of our graduating residents who might otherwise proceed directly to a general surgery practice choose to pursuit fellowship training because they feel that they have to either "finish" residency training or develop a niche market skill. Some general surgeons focus or limit their skill sets deliberately; some for the purpose of concentrating effort and study to improve outcomes, while possibly others may limit their skills to become "ineligible" to participate in some onerous task such as call. I would submit that there is no agreed upon definition of what a general surgeon is and/or what that person would or should do that would satisfy all parties involved.

Surg Clin N Am 90 (2010) ix–x
doi:10.1016/j.suc.2010.08.005
surgical.theclinics.com

Participation in armed conflict, in some respects, is liberating. Winston Churchill is credited with saying, "Nothing in life is so exhilarating as to have been shot at without result." That is something with which I might not entirely agree; however, I would suggest that being in a place in which one is shot at or mortared or rocketed most definitely does concentrate one's focus on what really is essential and what is not. Another liberating bit of the war environment is that it strips one of the millions of little ties to the everyday annoyances that we frequently regard as important matters. In short, participation in war very much re-defines perspective.

When Dr DeMeester graciously agreed to be our guest editor for this issue, we had a conversation about the topics we wished to include. As always, it was our goal to include topics that addressed the knowledge and practical needs of the general surgeon while maintaining the level of intellectual discipline of a specialist. I would submit that he and his colleagues have done an excellent job of achieving this. At the time we first discussed this the issues seemed to me to be more about covering a series of topics that many general surgeons needed to have knowledge of but were unlikely to directly participate in—but at that moment I was thinking in "peace-time" mode. Today, the topics appear every bit as useful and relevant to me but they also seem *essential*. Today I am thinking in "wartime" mode.

I can't say what the right balance is between general capabilities and specialty capabilities for all general surgeons. I can say that when one is 10,000 miles from home and you have a handful of surgeons and a small but highly motivated group of other health care professionals to care for horrifically wounded people, all knowledge seems essential no matter how you normally practice at home. Even if one is not as displaced as in war, one frequently may find oneself out of one's surgical comfort zone for other reasons. I am grateful to Dr DeMeester and his colleagues for giving us an excellent place to turn for clear and concise advice under such circumstances.

Ronald F. Martin, MD
Department of Surgery
Marshfield Clinic
1000 North Oak Avenue
Marshfield, WI 54449, USA

E-mail address:
martin.ronald@marshfieldclinic.org

Preface

Tracheobronchial, Pulmonary and Mediastinal Problems in General Thoracic Surgery

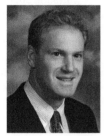

Steven R. DeMeester, MD
Guest Editor

In this issue of *Surgical Clinics of North America* there are 11 articles that encompass the spectrum of major thoracic issues that a general surgeon might encounter. Each article is written by a general thoracic surgeon, and each is aimed at the non-general thoracic surgeon such that the critical concepts for the evaluation, diagnosis and therapy of each condition are clearly detailed. One of the most common radiographic findings in ill patients is a pleural effusion, and management of the pleural space is expertly discussed by Dr Neil Christie. Likewise, pneumothorax and emphysema are frequently encountered clinical conditions that are reviewed by Dr Bryan Meyers. Dr Mary Maish beautifully discusses the diaphragm and associated problems, including hernia and eventration, while Dr Farzaneh Banki comprehensively reviews pre-operative pulmonary assessment in patients with thoracic surgical problems. The challenging topic of hemoptysis and pulmonary fungal infections is expertly discussed by Dr Brian Louie. Thoracic malignancy is covered from the evaluation of the solitary pulmonary nodule by Dr Ross Bremner, to tumors of the mediastinum and chest wall by Dr Wayne Hofstetter, and metastastectomy and non-resectional therapies for lung neoplasms by Dr Chrish Fernando. A thorough review of the options and strategies for endoscopic evaluation of the tracheobronchial tree and mediastinal lymph nodes is presented by Dr Tom Watson, while Dr Henning Gaissert provides valuable insights into the complexities of management of the compromised airway. Lastly, thoracic problems that are unique to the pediatric population are extensively reviewed by Dr Carl Backer. I am certain that you will find each article exceptionally well written and informative, and trust that this issue of *Surgical Clinics of North America* will

Surg Clin N Am 90 (2010) xi–xii
doi:10.1016/j.suc.2010.07.004
0039-6109/10/$ – see front matter © 2010 Elsevier Inc. All rights reserved.

surgical.theclinics.com

be on your short list of go-to references when thoracic surgical problems or issues are encountered in the practice of general surgery and daily care of patients.

Steven R. DeMeester, MD
University of Southern California
Keck School of Medicine
1520 San Pablo Street, Suite 4300
Los Angeles, CA 90033, USA

E-mail address:
Steven.Demeester@med.usc.edu

Management of Pleural Space: Effusions and Empyema

Neil A. Christie, MD

KEYWORDS

• Pleural effusion • Pleurodesis • Empyema • Thoracoscopy
• Fibrinolysis

Surgeons are commonly called on to evaluate patients with pleural effusions. This article discusses the normal anatomy, physiology, and pathophysiology of the pleural space. The signs and symptoms of pleural effusions as well as the evaluation of pleural effusions of unknown cause are also reviewed. Although pleural effusions can be seen in a host of medical disorders, the 2 main circumstances that the surgeon is involved with are with malignant pleural effusions and pleural sepsis and therefore the management of theses 2 entities is discussed in detail.

PLEURAL SPACE PHYSIOLOGY

The pleural space lies between the visceral and parietal pleura and consists of 2 opposed pleural surfaces separated by 10 to 20 μm of glycoprotein-rich fluid. The normal volume of pleural fluid is low, at approximately 10 mL (0.1–0.2 mL/kg body weight). Pleural fluid contains few cells under normal circumstances.[1] The normal pleura is a thin translucent membrane and consists of 5 layers: (1) the mesothelium (flattened mesothelial cells joined primarily by tight junctions); (2) submesothelial connective tissue; (3) a superficial elastic layer; (4) a second loose subpleural connective tissue layer rich in arteries, veins, and nerves; (5) a deep fibroelastic layer adherent to the underlying lung parenchyma, chest wall, and diaphragm or mediastinum.[2]

The parietal pleura derives its blood supply from branches of the intercostal arteries. The mediastinal pleura is supplied by the pericardiophrenic artery and the diaphragmatic pleura from the superior phrenic and musculophrenic arteries. The visceral pleura derives most of its blood supply from the bronchial arterial system.[2]

There exist naturally occurring pores, or stomata, in the caudal portion of the parietal pleura and lower mediastinal pleura that are capable of transferring particulate matter

Department of Cardiothoracic Surgery, University of Pittsburgh Medical Center, 5200 Centre Avenue, Suite 715, Pittsburgh, PA 15232, USA
E-mail address: christiena@upmc.edu

Surg Clin N Am 90 (2010) 919–934
doi:10.1016/j.suc.2010.07.003
0039-6109/10/$ – see front matter © 2010 Elsevier Inc. All rights reserved.

surgical.theclinics.com

and cells directly into lymphatic channels for removal. Most of the fluid that accumulates abnormally in the pleural space is derived from the lung through the visceral pleura and is absorbed primarily thorough the parietal pleura.[3] In disease states, excess production and/or decreased absorption of lymph is responsible for the generation of effusions.

Evaluation of Pleural Effusions

Causes of effusions are manifold. They can be classified as transudative with a low protein content (found in congestive heart failure, cirrhosis, nephrotic syndrome) or as exudative with a high protein content (found in cancer, infection, pulmonary emboli, pancreatitis, collagen vascular disease, drug-induced conditions, hemothorax, chylothorax).[4]

The clinical scenario is helpful in determining the cause of an effusion. Signs or symptoms of infection, history of malignancy, or associated medical diseases such as cardiac failure or kidney or liver disease can be helpful in determining the cause of an effusion.

Small pleural effusions are asymptomatic. Large pleural effusions can cause dyspnea, cough, and chest discomfort.

Effusions are generally seen on chest radiograph. Small pleural effusions may be evident as blunting of the costophrenic angle. A lateral decubitus film can confirm an effusion to be free flowing. Loculated effusions are harder to diagnose on a standard chest radiograph. Ultrasound can detect a loculated effusion and also determine an appropriate site for thoracentesis. A computed axial tomography (CAT) scan is useful in the evaluation of pleural effusions. It can determine the size and the location of the effusion and it also gives information regarding associated underlying parenchymal and pleural abnormalities.

Thoracentesis is useful to determine the cause of an effusion. Pleural fluid evaluation should include cytologic evaluation, culture, cell count, and differential and simultaneous pleural fluid and serum protein, glucose and lactate dehydrogenase (LDH) levels. Effusions are classified as exudative or transudative based on protein and LDH levels. (Exudate = pleural fluid protein/serum protein >0.5 and pleural fluid LDH/serum LDH >0.6.[4]) Malignant cells on cytologic evaluation indicate an underlying malignancy causing the effusion. Although the specificity of cytologic analysis is high, the sensitivity of a single cytologic evaluation can be as low as 50% and therefore often more invasive procedures may be required to diagnose an underlying malignancy, as discussed later.[5] Presence of an increased white blood cell count in the pleural fluid, particularly with a preponderance of neutrophils, may indicate pleural infection. Low pleural fluid glucose and pH are indicators of active pleural infection and the need for pleural drainage, as discussed in detail later.

A transudative effusion occurs most commonly secondary to congestive heart failure. Transudative effusions are generally managed by medical therapy for the underlying disease. Occasionally another intervention, such as pleurodesis, is required in cases refractory to maximal medical therapy. There are multiple causes for exudative effusions, but they are most commonly due to malignancy, infection, or pulmonary emboli. Overall, the 4 most common causes of pleural effusions in the United States are congestive heart failure, bacterial pneumonia, malignancy, and pulmonary emboli.[4]

Patients in whom a diagnosis of pleural effusion has not been ascertained after thoracentesis and CAT scan should undergo thoracoscopy and bronchosopy. Thoracoscopy allows direct pleural biopsy and also the potential for therapeutic intervention, including evacuation of the effusion either with or without pleurodesis.

The rest of this article focuses on the management of malignant pleural effusions, parapneumonic effusions, and empyema.

Malignant Pleural Effusions

Malignant pleural effusions cause dyspnea and decreased exercise tolerance, and may significantly affect a patient's quality of life. Approximately half of all patients with metastatic cancer develop a pleural effusion.[6] Drainage of pleural fluid with reexpansion of underlying lung can provide impressive relief of dyspnea and a significant improvement in the patient's overall sense of well-being.

Increased capillary permeability in patients with advanced cancer may result in increased pleural fluid production and simultaneously lymphatic obstruction by metastatic disease may result in decreased pleural fluid drainage. This imbalance between production and drainage of pleural fluid results in the development of a pleural effusion. Tumor cells in the pleural fluid also may contribute to pleural fluid accumulation by increasing the pleural osmotic pressure.[6]

Two general approaches exist for the management of symptomatic malignant pleural effusions: drainage and pleurodesis, or placement of a long-term pleural catheter for intermittent drainage at home. Thoracentesis alone should be offered as a therapeutic option only for patients in whom survival is expected to be short, or in the rare patient with a slowly reaccumulating malignant pleural effusion.

Pleurodesis is a treatment that aims to produce fibrosis of the pleura by chemical or mechanical means to obliterate the pleural space. The aim of pleurodesis in patients with malignant effusions is to prevent reaccumulation of the effusion after drainage, thereby permanently alleviating the associated symptoms. For successful pleurodesis to be achieved, the parietal and visceral pleura must be in apposition. In those patients in whom the lung incompletely reexpands after pleural fluid drainage pleurodesis is not successful. This condition is referred to as a trapped lung. Incomplete lung reexpansion after drainage of a malignant pleural effusion should be viewed as a contraindication to attempted sclerosis and is an indication to pursue alternative therapeutic options such as placement of a long-term indwelling pleural catheter. Furthermore, for pleurodesis to be successful, the patient must be able to mount an inflammatory response sufficient to fuse the pleural space. The use of antiinflammatory medications should be avoided in patients undergoing pleurodesis.

Sclerosing agents are instilled into the pleural space to induce pleurodesis. Multiple agents have been tried for this purpose. Shaw and Agarwal[6] reviewed studies comparing different sclerosants in an attempt to obtain pleurodesis in the Cochrane Database in 2009. Comparing different sclerosants, talc was found to be the most efficacious. The relative risk of nonrecurrence was 1.34 (95% confidence interval [CI] 1.16–1.55) in favor of talc compared with bleomycin, tetracycline, mustine, or tube drainage alone based on 10 randomized controlled studies involving 308 patients. In most studies the efficacy of talc was judged by radiographic evidence for the recurrence of an effusion or clinical need for repeat thoracenteses. Three studies compared talc with tetracycline with 103 participants and the relative risk of success favored talc at 1.32 (95% CI 1.10–1.72). Typically 5 g of talc are instilled into the pleural space to induce pleurosesis; either as a suspension in 50 to 100 mL normal saline via a chest tube, or via direct insufflation at thoracoscopy.

Some investigators have reported the development of acute lung injury after pleural talc instillation that can be associated with severe respiratory insufficiency and death. It seems to be related to the size of talc particles, and administration of filtered talc with uniform small particles is recommended.[7]

Currently most physicians base the decision of when to remove the chest drain after pleurodesis on volume of drainage as well as absence of fluid on a chest radiograph. There is a concern that a high volume of ongoing chest tube drainage impairs pleural apposition and pleural symphysis. Early chest tube removal is desirable because the average survival for patients with malignant pleural effusion is short. Earlier chest tube removal with the associated reduction in treatment times could also facilitate earlier return to chemotherapeutic agents.

One randomized trial evaluated the effectiveness of short-term versus longer-term drainage after talc slurry pleurodesis in patients with malignant pleural effusions.[8] Chest drains were removed at either 24 hours or 72 hours after talc slurry pleurodesis and the primary outcome measurement was freedom from pleural effusion recurrence at 1 month follow-up. These investigators performed pleurodesis with 4 g of talc when chest tube drainage was less than 150 mL/d. On average, there were 2 days between the insertion of chest drain and the instillation of sclerosant. The investigators found no difference in outcomes between chest tube removal at 24 hours versus 72 hours and an associated decreased length of stay (4 days in the early chest tube removal group vs 8 days in the other group). Pleural effusion recurrence was seen in 2 of 16 (13%) of the 24-hour group and 4 of 19 (21%) in the 72-hour group.

Another study evaluated the efficacy of short-term chest tube drainage versus standard chest tube drainage with tetracycline pleurodesis.[9] Generally it is recommended that pleurodesis be undertaken when chest tube drainage is less than 150 mL/d. In the standard group, pleurodesis with 1.5 g of tetracycline was performed when there was radiologic evidence of lung reexpansion and drainage volume less than 150 mL/d and chest tubes were removed when drainage was less than 150 mL/d. In the short-term group, tetracycline was instilled when the chest radiograph showed the lung to be expanded (usually at 24 hours) and the chest tube was removed the day following tetracycline instillation. A follow-up chest radiograph was obtained at 30 days to determine the response to sclerotherapy. A positive response was no fluid reaccumulation and nonresponders were defined as those with reaccumulation of greater than 50% of the original volume of fluid or those requiring fluid drainage within 1 month after treatment. Successful pleurodesis was seen in 80% and was the same in both groups. The duration of chest tube drainage was shorter in the study group at 2 days versus 7 days median in the standard group. A shorter duration of hospital stay was again shown without sacrificing the efficacy of pleurodesis.

There seems to be no justification for prolonged chest tube drainage either before or after instillation of sclerosant for pleurodesis. Although most physicians use at least 24 hours of chest tube drainage after pleurodesis to promote pleural symphysis, further delay in chest tube removal does not seem to be justified. Strategies such as rolling the patient after instillation of the sclerosing agent and larger chest tubes also have not been shown to offer any substantial advantages.[10]

Having established that talc seems to be the optimal agent for achieving pleurodesis, the next question is what is the optimal method for performing the procedure: following chest tube insertion with talc slurry instillation in the tube or by direct insufflation at the time of thoracoscopic pleural effusion drainage? Thoracoscopic and chest tube drainage can differ in several aspects, which may affect the efficacy of pleurodesis. The extent of drainage of an effusion before pleurodesis can affect the efficacy of pleurodesis and may vary depending whether this is performed via thoracoscopy or via a thoracostomy at the bedside. The distribution of the sclerosant over the pleural space may likewise differ depending on the method of instillation and may affect the likelihood of successful pleurodesis. The most effective sclerosant talc is often preferentially used in thoracoscopic pleurodesis and less frequently used in chest tube pleurodesis.

In the Cochrane review of 2 randomized studies of thoracoscopic versus chest tube pleurodesis, which included 112 participants, thoracoscopic pleurodesis was found to be more effective than chest tube pleurodesis, with a relative risk of non-recurrence of 1.19 (95% CI 1.04–1.36).[6] Another review of 5 randomized studies involving 145 patients compared thoracoscopic and bedside instillation of various sclerosants (tetracycline, bleomycin, talc, or mustine).[6] All but one study used talc as the sclerosant in the thoracoscopic arm. The relative risk of successful pleurodesis favored thoracoscopic instillation, with a relative risk of 1.68 (95% CI 1.35–2.10). This review must be interpreted with some caution secondary to the confounding effect of different sclerosants. There was no difference in the mortality among the participants who received thoracoscopic versus bedside instillation of talc. Data from these analyses suggest that thoracoscopic pleurodesis with talc may be the optimal technique for pleurodesis in patients with malignant pleural effusions.

More recently a prospective randomized trial of thoracoscopy with talc versus tube thoracostomy with talc slurry was published.[11] A total of 242 patients were treated with thoracoscopy and 240 were treated with a chest tube. The primary end point was freedom from pleural effusion recurrence. Only patients who achieved at least 90% initial lung reexpansion after drainage were included in the study. In the chest tube group, drainage occurred for 24 to 36 hours before instillation of the sclerosant and chest tubes were removed when the drainage was less than 150 mL/d. Of all patients evaluated, more than 90% lung reexpansion was achieved in 68% of patients treated with chest tubes and 73% of patients treated with thoracoscopy. Thirty-day mortality was high, at 20% in the patients treated with chest tube and 14% in the patients treated with thoracoscopy. Postprocedural respiratory failure and death was seen in 4% of patients treated with chest tube and 8% of patients undergoing thoracoscopy in this study. Overall 30-day successful outcome was not statistically significantly different between the 2 groups, at 78% with thoracoscopy and 71% with chest tube talc slurry instillation. The subgroup with primary lung or breast histopathology had a higher success rate with thoracoscopy (82% vs 67% in chest tube group).

Another prospective study, which was nonrandomized, compared outcomes with thoracoscopic talc pleurodesis versus tube thoracoscopy and talc slurry.[12] Patients at high risk for general anesthesia, and those with poor functional status or short life expectancy, were relegated to chest tube drainage, whereas the others were treated with thoracoscopy. Six grams of talc was used in both groups. Ninety-day outcomes were improved in the thoracoscopy group (88.3%) versus the chest tube group (69.9%). Patients with the tube thoracostomy reported a high incidence of pain with the procedure compared with the patients treated with thoracoscopy. Compared with the other study, no acute respiratory failure or early mortality was seen in either group. Overall survival was 7. 7 months, with a lower survival in the patients treated with chest tube (3.9 months) versus the patients treated with thoracoscopy (11.2 months).

Another large study reported outcomes of thoracoscopic talc pleurodesis in 611 patients treated between 1994 and 2003 with a mean follow-up of 319 days.[13] A total of 17.2% of patients died within 30 days of treatment and Karnofsky index (< 50%) and body mass index (calculated as weight in kilograms divided by the square of height in meters) of less than 25 kg/m^2 were predictive of an increased mortality. Radiographic improvement was seen in 68.6% and symptomatic improvement in 89.1%

immediately after drainage. Overall there were only 4 cases (0.6%) of empyema and 2 cases (0.3%) of procedurally related respiratory failure.

Although overall thoracoscopic drainage and pleurodesis seems to be the superior approach, the treatment of symptomatic malignant pleural effusions should be individualized by a patient's functional status and anticipated survival as well as the presence or absence of pleural apposition after drainage. Subjecting patients with poor functional status to thoracoscopy may result in procedure-related respiratory insufficiency and death.

An alternative method of palliating malignant pleural effusions involves the use of tunneled pleural catheters, which are left indwelling long-term. This is an option for patients who obtain symptomatic relief from the pleural drainage but do not show complete or near-complete lung expansion after pleural fluid drainage and are therefore not candidates for pleurodesis because pleural apposition is not obtained. Although prolonged pleural catheter drainage is useful in the management of malignant pleural effusion in the setting of incomplete lung reexpansion after drainage, it is also useful as a therapy for recurrent symptomatic malignant pleural effusion after a failed pleurodesis.

The pleurex catheter is a 15.5-French silicone catheter 66 cm long with fenestrations along the proximal 24 cm. On the distal end is a valve that prevents fluid or air from passing in either direction unless the catheter is accessed with a special drainage line. The pleural fluid is drained by inserting the access tip of the drainage line into the valve of the catheter and then draining into vacuum bottles. Insertion can potentially be performed as an outpatient. Seldinger technique is used to insert a wire into the pleural effusion at the anterior axillary line. A 5- to 8-cm chest wall tunnel is made and the catheter is pulled through the tunnel. After dilation of the wire tract, the catheter is fed through a peel-away sheath and into the pleural space. Given that the presence of a malignant pleural effusion usually precludes cure and objectives are palliative, an advantage of indwelling pleural catheters is that they can cause immediate and long-term relief of symptoms and also minimize or avoid hospitalization altogether.

One large study reviewed the outcomes of 250 tunneled pleural catheters placed in 223 patients (19 patients had bilateral catheters and 8 had repeat ipsilateral procedures).[14] Symptom control was complete in 38.8% of patients and partial in 50%. In 10 patients (4%) there was a failure to successfully place the catheter. Following successful catheter placement, no further ipsilateral procedure was required in 90% of cases. The catheters were placed in a procedure room as an outpatient. Catheters were drained 3 times per week at home.

Most patients had lung cancer (37%), breast cancer (20%), or mesothelioma (12%). There was no difference in symptom control based on primary tumor type. The size of residual effusion at 2 weeks after catheter placement significantly corresponded with the degree of symptom control.

A total of 46% of catheters stayed in until the time of patient death and overall median survival was 144 days. Thirty-day and 1-year mortality were 13% and 84%, respectively. Spontaneous pleurodesis occurred in 43% of patients, allowing removal of the catheter. The catheter was removed once the volume of drainage was less than 50 mL on 3 sequential drainage attempts and fluid reaccumulation was not detected on chest radiograph. In these patients the median duration of catheter drainage was 56 days. The only factor predicting the likelihood of spontaneous pleurodesis was size of residual pleural effusion at less than 20% of original at 2 weeks after placement of catheter with a 57% rate of spontaneous pleurodesis (vs a 25% rate in patients with larger residual effusions).

Although 90% of patients required no reinterventions, 10% required reintervention: repeat catheter placement in 9 patients; thoracentesis in 6 patients; chest tube placement in 5 patients; and pleural fibrinolysis in 4 patients. Fifteen catheters were removed for reasons other than spontaneous pleurodesis: empyema in 5 patients; subcutaneous emphysema in 1 patient; accidental dislodgement in 3 patients; and extrapleural placement in 1 patient.

Complications included unsuccessful placement in 4%; symptomatic loculated effusion in 8.4%; asymptomatic loculation in 4%; empyema in 3.2%; subcutaneous air in 2.4%; cellulitis in 1.6%; and accidental dislodgement in 1.6%.

Empyemas were treated with hospitalization with intravenous antibiotics and continuous pleural drainage via pleural catheter with either thrombolysis or additional chest drains used as needed for loculated collections of fluid.

The investigators did speculate that the lack of complete resolution of symptoms was likely due to coincidental factors such as chronic obstructive pulmonary disease, lymphangitic carcinomatosis, and malignant airway obstruction.

Another study looked at effectiveness of pleural catheter drainage in a subset of patients who would be considered good candidates for pleurodesis.[15] These patients had an estimated survival greater than 90 days and less than 20% residual pleural effusion after drainage (not a trapped lung). Symptomatic improvement was seen in all patients (67% complete and 33% partial). Spontaneous pleurodesis occurred in 76 of 109 patients (70%) at a mean of 90 days. Of the remaining patients, catheters stayed in until death in 19%. Three patients developed empyema (4.6%).

Another study compared the effectiveness of chronic indwelling catheter versus doxycycline instillation via tube thoracostomy in patients with symptomatic malignant pleural effusion.[16] Six of 28 patients (21%) treated with doxycycline pleurodesis had recurrence of the pleural fluid. Twelve of 91 patients with an indwelling catheter (13%) had recurrence of fluid or blockage of the catheter. Symptomatic control after treatment was identical in both groups. A total of 46% of the 91 pleural catheters achieved spontaneous pleurodesis at a median of 27 days. Hospitalization was 1 day for the catheter group and 6.5 days for the doxycycline group. Degree of pain experienced in the 2 groups was similar and overall survival was poor, but similar in both groups (90 days in the patients treated with chest tube and 87 days in the patients treated with pleural catheter). The investigators concluded that a chronic indwelling catheter is an effective treatment option for the management of patients with symptomatic recurrent malignant pleural effusion, and is associated with a shorter hospitalization and the option for outpatient management.

Although long-term pleural catheter placement should be considered the treatment of choice for management of symptomatic malignant pleural effusion in patients with an entrapped lung, controversy remains as to the role in patients thought to be appropriate candidates for standard pleurodesis procedures. Factors influencing this decision may include patient preference, outpatient support for intermittent home drainage, and local institutional expertise.

There are no randomized trials on the role of pleurectomy or decortication in the management of malignant pleural effusions. A review of 5 case series covering 260 patients revealed a perioperative mortality up to 12.5% and a high incidence of prolonged postoperative air leak, at 10% to 20%.[10] This review included patients with mesothelioma and patients with other malignant diseases in which tumor debulking and decortication were part of the procedure. In some patients, decortication was performed when the lung was seen to be entrapped. Except for select patients with a primary pleural tumor (such as mesothelioma) in whom local chemotherapy may be applied, or in cases of indolent metastatic tumors confined to the thorax such as thymic tumors, this aggressive surgical approach should not be considered. In the general group of patients with metastatic cancer and symptomatic malignant pleural effusions who are debilitated with limited life expectancy, pleurectomy and decortication are generally not recommended given the significant associated major morbidity and mortality.

PLEURAL SPACE INFECTION

Infection of the pleura and pleural space is most often the result of an infection arising in the ipsilateral lung (pneumonia, lung abscess, or bronchiectasis). However, the associated pulmonary consolidation may be minimal. Despite the widespread use of antibiotics for respiratory tract infections, pleural empyema still occurs. At least 40% of all patients hospitalized with pneumonia have an associated pleural effusion.[17] In the United States, empyema is seen in about 60,000 patients annually, with a mortality of 15%.[17] Other causes of pleural sepsis are after lung surgery, trauma, esophageal perforation, and transdiaphragmatic spread of intraabdominal infection. Of all patients with pneumonia who develop a pleural effusion, only a few require intervention for a complicated parapneumonic effusion or an empyema. A parapneumonic effusion refers to any effusion secondary to pneumonia or a lung abscess. An empyema refers to frank pus in the pleural space. Complex parapneumonic effusions and empyema are more common at the extremes of age.

The development of a parapneumonic effusion occurs in 3 clinically relevant stages that represent a continuous spectrum. When the pleura is faced with an infectious organism, it responds with edema and exudation of proteins and neutrophils and a rapid influx of fluid into the pleural space. This process translates in to the classically observed exudative pleural effusion. In the exudative stage the increased rate of pleural fluid formation results from increased permeability of pleural capillaries and the pleural mesothelium. Mesothelial cells play a pivotal role in the development of the intrapleural inflammatory cascade by acting as phagocytes and triggering an inflammatory response when activated by bacteria. The resultant release of chemokines, cytokines, oxidants, and proteases contributes directly to the inflammation as well as secondarily by recruiting neutrophils and mononuclear phagocytes to the pleural space.[17]

The exudative stage is characterized by a sterile exudate secondary to increased permeability of the visceral pleura. The rapidity and extent of progression depends on the type and virulence of the organism, the patient's host defenses, and the timing and effectiveness of antibiotic treatment.[17] Initially, in the uncomplicated parapneumonic effusion, the pleural fluid has a pH greater than 7.20, glucose levels in the normal range and LDH levels less than 3 times the upper limit of normal. Most patients with uncomplicated parapneumonic effusions respond to antibiotics alone. If the infectious injury is promptly resolved, healing typically occurs with few permanent sequelae.

Untreated exudative effusions may develop into fibrinopurulent effusions or complex parapneumonic effusions. The fibrinopurulent stage represents pleural infection with the deposition of fibrin on visceral and parietal pleural membranes and the formation of loculations. Ongoing phagocytosis and cell lysis result in pleural fluid that has a pH less than 7.20, LDH levels more than 3 times normal, and low glucose. Characteristic of the fibrinopurulent stage of pleural sepsis is a disturbance in the physiologic equilibrium between clotting and fibrinolysis within the pleural space. Deposition of fibrin along pleural membranes may occlude lymphatic stomata, thereby decreasing the reabsorption capacity of the pleural space for fluid causing a further increase in the pleural effusion. Pleural surfaces become coated with fibrin and fibrin strands, which results in adhesions and loculations within the pleural space. This process complicates pleural fluid drainage by preventing the free flow of pleural fluid.[17] This second stage is characterized by a positive Gram stain and/or positive microbial cultures. A complicated parapneumonic effusion requires at least pleural catheter drainage and possibly surgical intervention.

A complex parapneumonic effusion progresses to a pleural empyema when the concentration of leukocytes becomes sufficient to form frank pus as characterized by viscous, whitish-yellow turbid to opaque pleural fluid. Empyema fluid consists of fibrin, cellular debris, and viable or dead bacteria.

The third and final stage of pleural infection is the organizing phase. The organization stage occurs with the influx of fibroblasts into the pleural space and formation of inelastic pleural peel with dense fibrous septations. Fibroblasts grow into the pleural space from both the visceral and parietal pleura. During this fibrotic response the pleural space may become focally or massively obliterated and be accompanied by the formation of dense fibrous adhesions. This process eventually results in a thick pleural peel that restricts chest mechanics and often necessitates a surgical decortication to address restrictive impairment.[17] Animal research suggests an important role for transforming growth factor β in the development of pleural fibrosis.[18]

Presentation of patients with empyema may vary depending on the underlying bacterial cause. Patients with aerobic infections tend to be more acutely ill and the presentation is similar to pneumonia, followed by a nonresolving pneumonia picture with pleuritic chest pain, persistent fever spikes, and failure to improve on appropriate antibiotic therapy. Elderly individuals, immunocompromised patients, and those with anaerobic infections can have a more indolent course and may present with weight loss, cough, fever, and anemia.[19] The pleural effusions are generally evident on chest radiographs. Lateral decubitus films may help to assess loculations. Ultrasound can show the presence of loculations and can also be used to guide pleural drainage, particularly in loculated effusions.[20] CAT scan is helpful to best delineate the size and location of pleural collections, the presence of loculations, as well as the status of the underlying lung parenchyma.[21]

Initial antibiotic coverage of patients with parapneumonic effusions is generally dictated by treatment guidelines for pneumonia and altered according to blood and pleural fluid microbial cultures and sensitivities. Empiric anaerobic antibiotic coverage may be advised because there may be an anaerobic infection, which is generally not so amenable to cultures as anaerobes. Patients with nosocomial empyema need adequate gram-negative coverage. Vancomycin may be added for suspected methicillin-resistant infection. Reported bacteriology of pleural sepsis varies significantly between community acquired and nosocomial infections.[22] Early appropriate antibiotic therapy represents the cornerstone of therapy for pneumonia and parapneumonic effusion.

Minimal size free-flowing effusions may be observed without a diagnostic aspiration because the risk of a complicated course is remote. However, all but the very small free-flowing effusions should be aspirated for diagnostic purposes. Pleural fluid should be evaluated for cytology, cell count, Gram stain, and culture as well as pH, LDH, glucose, and protein.

Uncomplicated parapneumonic exudative effusions that are of small volume and free flowing without loculations with a negative Gram stain, pH greater than 7.20, and negative cultures are usually inflammatory in nature and have no detectable bacterial pathogens. Most of these resolve with antibiotic therapy for the underlying pneumonia and can therefore be observed without formal drainage.[17]

However, early drainage of pleural fluid becomes necessary when a parapneumonic effusion advances beyond the exudative stage to the fibrinopurulent stage and becomes a complicated parapneumonic effusion. Indications for immediate drainage are large effusions (>half the hemithorax), effusions with loculations, pH less than 7.20, positive Gram stain or culture and low glucose levels. The presence of frank pus on aspiration, which constitutes an empyema, is also an indication for immediate drainage.[17]

Options for drainage include: multiple thoracenteses; tube thoracostomy (± intrapleural fibrinolytics); thoracoscopic drainage; thoracotomy and drainage (± decortication); and chronic open drainage. Choice of drainage is dependent on the viscosity of the pleural fluid, location, volume and extent of loculations, and the general condition of the patient.

Multiple thoracenteses are generally not recommended. One study showed patients required an average of 7.7 aspirates and had a hospital stay of 31 days.[23]

Tube thoracostomy is generally performed with a size 24 to 28 French chest tube placed in a dependent area (usually the posterior costophrenic recess). Sometimes ultrasound guidance can be used to guide placement of smaller tubes. The benefit of image guidance for smaller tubes may be offset by the greater propensity of the smaller tubes to clot.

Complicated parapneumonic effusions and empyema are characterized by a procoagulant state within the pleural space, which results in the progressive development of dense layers of fibrin and loculations, as discussed earlier. These complex loculated effusions may not be adequately drained with a simple tube thoracostomy alone. Options for treatment include tube thoracostomy with subsequent administration of fibrinolytic agents thorough the tube, or surgical thoracoscopic drainage with mechanical disruption of adhesions and complete evacuation of thick inflammatory debris.

One could theorize that the administration of intrapleural fibrinolytics early in the fibrinopurulent phase could prevent loculations and promote pleural drainage. Intrapleural instillation of fibrinolytic agents theoretically could dissolve fibrinous clots and adhesions and prevent pleural loculations. The hope of intrapleural fibrinolytics would be to enhance pleural fluid drainage via tube thoracostomy and reduce the need for thoracoscopic surgical drainage. Use of fibrinolytic agents is appealing because the most common reason for failure of pleural drainage among patients with an appropriately positioned catheter is occlusion of the catheter by viscous fibrin-rich fluid and cellular debris, or the formation of fibrin strands that form pleural loculations that sequester pleural fluid and prevent it from reaching the chest tube. Side effects are minimal with rare reports of fever and bleeding.[24]

Streptokinase, urokinase, and tissue plasminogen activator are 3 fibrinolytic agents that have been widely used via chest tube instillation in the treatment of loculated parapneumonic effusion and empyema. Streptokinase is usually administered as 250,000 IU in 100 to 200 mL saline daily for up to 7 days. Urokinase is usually administered as 100,000 IU in 100 mL saline daily up to 3 days. Tissue plasminogen activator is usually administered as 10 to 25 mg twice daily up to 3 days. Drains should be clamped for 2 to 8 hours following the administration of the fibrinolytic. Tissue plasminogen activator provides fibrinolytic activity without the antigenicity of streptokinase.[17]

Tuncozgur and colleagues[25] looked at fibrinolytic versus saline instillation via chest tube in 49 patients. They found a significantly lower decortication rate (60% vs 29%) and shorter duration of hospitalization (14 vs 21 days) with the addition of intrapleural fibrinolysis as well as a greater volume of chest tube drainage (1.8 L vs 0.8 L).

A single-center randomized placebo-controlled study by Diacon and colleagues[26] reported that intrapleural streptokinase resulted in faster resolution of infection and reduced need for surgery (13.6% vs 45.5%) and improved outcomes in patients with complex parapneumonic effusions and empyema.

Another prospective study by Misthos and colleagues[27] investigated tube thoracostomy versus tube thoracostomy and streptokinase. Tube thoracostomy alone was successful in 67% of cases. Instillation of streptokinase led to a favorable outcome in 87% and significantly shortened hospital stay, mortality, and rate of surgical intervention.

Davies and colleagues[28] compared fibrinolysis versus saline control in the second to fifth hospital day in 24 patients with tube thoracostomy for empyema. These investigators looked at volume of drainage and improvement in chest radiographs. Fibrinolytics caused an increased rate of fluid drainage and greater improvement on chest radiograph. No bleeding complications were seen. Three patients in the control group and none in the fibrinolytic group required surgical drainage.

Bouros and colleagues[29] compared fibrinolytics with saline control in 31 patients. Fibrinolytic patients had a larger volume of drainage and higher rates of successful chest tube drainage (87% vs 25%) compared with saline control patients. Two patients treated with fibrinolytic therapy required surgical drainage and 12 patients with saline crossed over to fibrinolytic therapy, with 6 of 12 ultimately requiring surgical drainage.

Tokuda and colleagues[30] published a meta-analysis of all the major placebo-controlled studies on intrapleural fibrinolysis, and although they showed a trend toward improved survival and a decreased need for surgical interventions, the differences failed to be statistically significant.

Twenty-five small uncontrolled clinical trials reported on the safety and efficacy of intrapleural fibrinolytics in decreasing the need for surgical intervention. Aggregate mean success rate in avoiding surgery was 82% for streptokinase and 84% for urokinase. When treatment failure was considered as surgical intervention, fibrinolytics decreased the risk of this outcome (relative risk 0.63; 0.46–0.85).[31] However, there was discordance between the early studies and the more recent randomized control study by Maskell reported later.

The largest prospective multicenter double-blind controlled MIST trial (Multicenter Intrapleural Sepsis Trial) on the role of intrapleural streptokinase for pleural infection was reported in 2005.[32] In this large trial multicenter patients received either streptokinase (250,000 IU twice daily for 3 days) via chest tube or saline placebo. Primary end points of the study were death and need for surgical drainage. A total of 454 patients with pleural pus, pH less than 7.20, or bacterial invasion of the pleural space were randomized to chest tube drainage or tube drainage and streptokinase. The proportion of patients who died or needed surgery at 3 months was similar between streptokinase and control (31% vs 27%, $P = .43$). No differences in mortality, rate of surgery, radiographic outcomes, or length of hospital stay were shown. This study did not substantiate the role of streptokinase in pleural infections. The investigators speculated that the increased viscosity of pleural pus in patients with empyema may be related to high concentrations of DNA resulting from breakdown of phagocytes, bacteria, and other intrapleural cells and that DNase in addition to fibrinolytics may be more effective than fibrinolytics alone.

Antibiotics alone remain the standard for uncomplicated parapneumonic effusions. For free-flowing complicated parapneumonic effusion or unilocular empyema, tube thoracostomy or percutaneous catheter drainage remain the standard of care. No high-grade evidence from a large-scale randomized controlled study exists to support the administration of fibrinolytic therapy and so it should not be routinely used for all such patients. However, critics have pointed out that the duration of therapy and other methodologic issues in the randomized trial may have contributed to the failure of lytic therapy to show a significant advantage. In many centers lytic therapy is the mainstay of management for early empyema and substantially reduces the burden of patients needing surgical decortication.

Surgical drainage via thoracoscopy is the optimal therapy in patients who fail chest tube drainage, such as patients with an organized empyema with highly viscous pleural fluid and a trapped lung who experience failure of a tube thoracostomy to yield reexpansion of the lung.

Surgical therapy is also optimal primary therapy in patients who present with multi-locular complex parapneumonic effusions and empyema. However, there does seem to be a place for selective use of fibrinolytics in the early management of patients who fail drainage with appropriate sized chest tubes if reasons exist to avoid definitive surgical drainage. Fibrinolytic therapy may therefore be considered in poor surgical candidates who fail chest tube drainage, or in those who require a period of medical stabilization before surgery is performed, as well as in centers where surgical facilities are limited. Patient factors, local expertise, and surgical availability to a certain extent dictate the initial choice between tube thoracoscopy and fibrinolytics or thoracoscopy. Surgical drainage via thoracoscopy may be performed following fibrinolytics if complete drainage is not achieved.

As noted earlier, thoracoscopy seems to be the optimal treatment option for patients with an incompletely drained thick unilocular collection with incomplete lung expansion, as well as in patients with multiloculated parapneumonic effusion and empyema because loculations can be broken down, thick pleural fluid and debris completely evacuated, the pleural space can be extensively lavaged, and chest tubes can be carefully placed. However, the alternative to early surgical drainage via thora-coscopy is tube thoracostomy in all patients (± fibrinolytic therapy) and reserving surgery for those patients who cannot be managed by nonsurgical means.

Several small retrospective and unblinded prospective studies suggest that thora-coscopy is superior to tube thoracostomy with fibrinolytics, with the need for thora-cotomy halved.[33–35] In the only prospective randomized controlled trial of fibrinolytic therapy versus thoracoscopy for empyema, Wait and coworkers[36] randomly assigned 20 patients with complicated multiloculated parapneumonic and empyema to strepto-kinase (250,000 IU daily for 3 days) via tube thoracostomy or immediate thoracoscopic drainage. Thoracoscopy had a higher treatment success rate (91% vs 44%), lower duration of chest tube drainage (5.8 vs 9.8 days), and a shorter hospital stay (8.7 vs 12.8 days). This study supports the preferred approach of primary thoracoscopic drainage in patients presenting with multilocular collections, provided that they are suitable candidates for surgical intervention.

Decortication is a procedure in the chronic organizing phase that aims to restore chest mechanics by removing a restrictive fibrotic peel when the underlying lung is unable to expand (ie, trapped lung) because of the establishment of a thick inflamma-tory coat. The procedure entails the excision of all the fibrous tissue from the pleura to permit lung reexpansion.[37] Decortication relies on lung elasticity to fill the cavity. Lung constriction after empyema can reduce lung perfusion by 20% to 25% on the involved side. If after 6 months the pleura remains thickened and the patient's pulmonary func-tion is sufficiently reduced to limit activities, decortication should be considered. The pulmonary function of patients who undergo decortication can increase significantly. Decortication can improve lung perfusion and improve vital capacity from 62% up to 80% and the FEV_1 (forced expiratory volume after 1 second) from 50% to 69%.

Despite the improvement in volumes, the affected lung still remains impaired. It remains a procedure with significant morbidity and a reported mortality of up to 10% so the patient must be fit enough for a major intervention.[35] Some investigators report that pleural thickening may resolve over time and recommend deferring decortication for up to 6 months.[38] For asymptomatic patients in whom the sepsis has cleared, the benefit of the procedure is not proved and observation is warranted.

When managing patients with pleural infections in the acute stage, decortication should be considered only for control of pleural sepsis and is rarely required. Generally in the acute phase, lung expansion is possible with thoracoscopic drainage because pleural encasement is not fibrotic. Failure of reexpansion of the lung in the acute phase may be more often secondary to problems of the underlying lung parenchyma that would not be responsive to pleurectomy. It should be applied in the acute phase only if the pleural sepsis cannot be controlled in any other way; debilitated patients may be better managed with open thoracosotomy.

For patients in whom sepsis cannot be controlled acutely with thoracoscopic drainage, and in whom decortication is not appropriate, then window thoracostomy may be performed. Open thoracostomy may be the procedure of choice if there is a permanent supply of causative organisms as a result of bronchopleural fistula or if there is a space issue such as in a postpneumonectomy empyema. Postpneumonectomy empyema is a result of bronchopleural fistula in 80% to 100% of cases, with a mortality of 5% to 35%.[39,40] From 2% to 10% of pneumonectomies are followed by the development of a bronchopleural fistula.[39]

Open thoracostomy may be performed as a permanent procedure, or as a preliminary procedure before a more definitive treatment.

Definitive treatment after open thoracostomy is a procedure for obliterating the pleural space and this can be accomplished by one of 2 approaches. Thoracoplasty entails diminishing the distance between the lung parenchyma and chest wall by collapsing the roof of the chest wall.[41] The other option is to fill the space with transposition of viable tissue such as omentum or skeletal muscle. It can be performed as a primary procedure to manage an empyema space or as a staged procedure some months after an open thoracostomy. If an empyema is associated with a bronchopleural fistula, that also needs to be addressed. Operative closure of the bronchial stump can be performed via the previous thoracotomy or transsternally using a transpericardial approach.[42] Amputation of the airway stump and, on occasion, even carinal resections have been reported.[43] For chronic leaks from the peripheral lung (not the central airway) caused by destruction of the barrier function of the pleural space, placement of vascularized tissue and pleural space obliteration alone should be adequate.

SUMMARY

Pleural effusions can occur because of a host of underlying problems. Initial evaluation includes taking a careful medical history, performing a thoracentesis and pleural fluid analysis, and CAT scan imaging. If the cause of the effusion is still not clear after these evaluations and the effusion persists, then a thoracoscopic evaluation with pleural biopsy is generally indicated.

Malignant pleural effusions are ideally treated with thoracoscopy and talc pleurodesis. In patients with poor functional status, tube thoracoscopy and subsequent pleurodesis with sclerosant instillation via the chest tube may be better tolerated. Patients with an entrapped lung are optimally treated with a semipermanent indwelling pleural catheter.

Patients with pneumonia and associated pleural effusion should also be evaluated with thoracentesis. Presence of loculations, or pleural fluid analysis showing bacteria on Gram stain or culture, low glucose or low pH, and frank pus are all indications for immediate drainage. Nonloculated parapneumonic effusion and empyema may be adequately treated with a tube thoracoscopy, but loculated effusions, or those inadequately drained with a chest tube, are best treated with thoracoscopic drainage or a trial of lytic therapy. The fundamental principle of therapy is to eliminate residual space between the pleural surfaces. Existence or lack of dead space within the pleural cavity is a decisive factor influencing outcomes because no effective infection control can be expected in the presence of an active cavity. In select symptomatic patients who have persistent lung entrapment after treatment of an empyema with an associated restrictive defect, thoracotomy and decortication may be indicated to improve pulmonary function.

REFERENCES

1. Sahn SA. State of the art, the pleura. Am Rev Respir Dis 1988;138(1):184–234.
2. Wang NS. Anatomy of the pleura. Clin Chest Med 1998;19(2):229–40.
3. Wang N. The preformed stomas connecting the pleural cavity and the lymphatics in the parietal pleura. Am Rev Respir Dis 1975;111:12–20.
4. Rusch VW. Pleural effusions: benign and malignant. In: Patterson GA, Cooper JD, Deslauriers J, et al, editors. Pearson's thoracic and esophageal surgery. 3rd edition. Philadelphia: Churchill Livingstone; 2008. p. 1042–54. [Chapter 85].
5. Heffner J, Klein J. Recent advances in the diagnosis and management of malignant pleural effusions. Mayo Clin Proc 2008;83(2):235–50.
6. Shaw P, Agarwal R. Pleurodesis for malignant pleural effusions. Cochrane Database Syst Rev 2009;1:CD0002916. DOI:10.1002/14651858.CD0002916.pub2.
7. Maskell NA, Lee YC, Gleeson FV, et al. Randomised trials describing lung inflammation after pleurodesis with talc of varying particle size. Am J Respir Crit Care Med 2004;170:377–82.
8. Goodman A, Davies C. Efficacy of short-term versus long-term chest tube drainage following talc slurry pleurodesis in patients with malignant pleural effusions: a randomized trial. Lung Cancer 2006;54:51–5.
9. Villanueva AG, Gray AW, Shahian DM, et al. Efficacy of short term versus long term tube thoracostomy drainage before tetracycline pleurodesis in the treatment of malignant pleural effusions. Thorax 1994;49(1):23–5.
10. Tan C, Sedrakyan A, Browne J, et al. The evidence on the effectiveness of management for malignant pleural effusion: a systematic review. Eur J Cardiothorac Surg 2006;29:829–38.
11. Dresler C, Olak J, Herndon J, et al. Phase III intergroup study of talc poudrage vs talc slurry sclerosis for malignant pleural effusion. Chest 2005;127:909–15.
12. Stefani A, Natali P, Casali C, et al. Talc poudrage versus talc slurry in the treatment of malignant pleural effusion. A prospective comparison study. Eur J Cardiothorac Surg 2006;30:827–32.
13. Steger V, Mika U, Toomes H, et al. Who gains most? A 10-year experience with 611 thoracoscopic talc pleurodeses. Ann Thorac Surg 2007;83:1940–5.
14. Tremblay A, Michaud G. Single-center experience with 250 tunneled pleural catheter insertions for malignant pleural effusion. Chest 2006;129(2):362–8.
15. Tremblay A, Mason C, Michaud G. Use of tunneled catheters for malignant pleural effusions in patients fit for pleurodesis. Eur Respir J 2007;30:759–62.
16. Putnam JB, Light R, Rodriguez RM, et al. A randomized comparison of indwelling pleural catheter and doxycycline pleurodesis in the management of malignant pleural effusions. Cancer 1999;86:1992–9.

17. Koegelenberg CF, Diacon AH, Bolliger CT. Parapneumonic pleural effusion and empyema. Respiration 2008;75:241–50.
18. Sasse SA, Jadus MR, Kukes GD. Pleural fluid transforming factor beta-one correlates with pleural fibrosis in experimental empyema. Am J Respir Crit Care Med 2003;168:700–5.
19. Light RW. Parapneumonic effusions and empyema. Proc Am Thorac Soc 2006;3:75–80.
20. Tsai TH, Yang PC. Ultrasound in the diagnosis and management of pleural disease. Curr Opin Pulm Med 2003;9:282–90.
21. Aquino SL, Webb WR, Gushiken BJ. Pleural exudates and transudates: diagnosis with contrast-enhanced CT. Radiology 1994;192:803–8.
22. Chapman SJ, Davies RJ. Recent advances in parapneumonic effusions and empyema. Curr Opin Pulm Med 2004;10:299–304.
23. Simmers TA, Jie C, Sie B. Minimally invasive treatment of thoracic empyema. Thorac Cardiovasc Surg 1999;47:77–81.
24. Bouros D, Tzouvelekis A, Antoniou KM, et al. Intrapleural fibrinolytic therapy for pleural infection. Pulm Pharmacol Ther 2007;20:616–26.
25. Tuncozgur B, Ustunsoy H, Sirikoz MC, et al. Intrapleural urokinase in the management of parapneumonic empyema: a randomized controlled trial. Int J Clin Pract 2001;55:658–60.
26. Diacon AH, Theron J, Schuurmans MM, et al. Intrapleural streptokinase for empyema and complicated parapneumonic effusions. Am J Respir Crit Care Med 2004;170:49–53.
27. Misthos P, Sepsa E, Konstantinou M, et al. Early use of intrapleural fibrinolytics in the management of postpneumonic empyema. A prospective study. Eur J Cardiothorac Surg 2005;28:599–603.
28. Davies RJ, TRaill ZC, Gleeson FV. Randomized controlled trial of intrapleural streptokinase in community acquired pleural infections. Thorax 1997;52:416–21.
29. Bouros D, Schiza S, Tzanakis N, et al. Intrapleural urokinase versus normal saline in the treatment of complicated parapneumonic effusions and empyema. A randomized, double-blind study. Am J Respir Crit Care Med 1999;159:37–42.
30. Tokuda Y, Matsushima D, Stein GH, et al. Intrapleural fibrinolytic agents for empyema and complicated parapneumonic effusions: a meta-analysis. Chest 2006;129:783–90.
31. Cameron R, Davies HR. Intrapleural fibrinolytic therapy versus conservative management in the treatment of adult parapneumonic effusions and empyema. Cochrane Database Syst Rev 2008;2:CD0023112.
32. Maskell NA, Davies CW, Nunn AJ, et al. U.K. Controlled trial of intrapleural streptokinase for pleural infection. N Engl J Med 2005;352:865–74.
33. Cassina PC, Hauser M, Hillejan L, et al. Video-assisted thoracoscopy in the treatment of pleural empyema: stage-based management and outcome. J Thorac Cardiovasc Surg 1999;117:234–8.
34. Silen ML, Naunheim KS. Thoracoscopic approach to the management of empyema thoracis: indications and results. Chest Surg Clin N Am 1996;6:491–9.
35. Pothula V, Krellenstein DJ. Early aggressive surgical management of parapneumonic empyemas. Chest 1994;105:832–6.
36. Wait MA, Sharma S, Hohn J, et al. A randomized trial of empyema therapy. Chest 1997;111:1548–51.
37. Thurer RJ. Decortication in thoracic empyema: indications and surgical technique. Chest Surg Clin N Am 1996;6:461–90.

38. Neff CC, van Sonnenberg E, Lawson DW, et al. CT follow-up of empyemas: pleural peels resolve after percutaneous catheter drainage. Radiology 1990; 176:195–7.
39. Zaheer S, Allen MS, Cassivi SD, et al. Postpneumonectomy empyema: results after the Claggett procedure. Ann Thorac Surg 2006;82:279–86.
40. Athanassiadi K, Kalvrouziotis K, Bellenis I. Bronchopleural fistula after pneumo-nectomy: a major challenge. Acta Chir Hung 1999;38(1):5–7.
41. Icard P, LeRochais JP, Rabut B, et al. Andrews thoracoplasty as a treatment of post-pneumonectomy empyema: experience in 23 cases. Ann Thorac Surg 1999;68:1159–63.
42. De laRiviere AB, Defauw JJ, Knaepen PJ, et al. Transsternal closure of broncho-pleural fistula after pneumonectomy. Ann Thorac Surg 1997;64:954–7.
43. Athanassiadi K, Vassilikos K, Misthos P, et al. Late postpneumonectomy broncho-pleural fistula. Thorac Cardiovasc Surg 2004;52:298–301.

Pneumothorax, Bullous Disease, and Emphysema

Victor van Berkel, MD, PhD[a], Elbert Kuo, MD, MPH[b],
Bryan F. Meyers, MD, MPH[c],*

KEYWORDS

- Pneumothorax • Bullous disease • Emphysema
- Pulmonary conditions

This article discusses several conditions that are distinct entities but share the common thread of abnormal lung parenchyma that regularly leads to patient referral for surgical consideration. The article summarizes key aspects of the 3 conditions and provides advice and recommendations for evaluation and treatment based on published reports in the medical literature.

PNEUMOTHORAX
Definition

A pneumothorax is defined as air in the pleural space, between the parietal and visceral pleura. This condition may be caused by trauma or underlying lung disease, but sometimes happens spontaneously without obvious cause. When a pneumothorax develops, there is loss of the negative intrapleural pressure that is needed for lung inflation, and the lung on the affected side collapses and cannot expand properly. This collapse leads to a ventilation-perfusion mismatch because there is continued perfusion of a poorly ventilated lung. Arterial hypoxemia can occur with 50% collapse of the lung. If there is a continued air leak with increasing positive intrapleural pressure, this can lead to a tension pneumothorax and can lead to compromise of venous return to the heart, decreasing cardiac output, and causing hemodynamic collapse.

Causes

Pneumothorax can be spontaneous, traumatic, or iatrogenic. Primary spontaneous pneumothorax typically occurs in young, healthy, tall, thin, male smokers and is

[a] Division of Cardiothoracic Surgery, Department of Surgery, University of Louisville School of Medicine, Louisville, KY, USA
[b] Heart and Lung Institute, St Joseph's Hospital and Medical Center, Phoenix, AZ, USA
[c] Division of Cardiothoracic Surgery, Department of Surgery, Washington University School of Medicine, Barnes-Jewish Hospital Plaza Street, Saint Louis, MO 63110-1013, USA
* Corresponding author. One Barnes-Jewish Hospital Plaza Street, 3108 Queeny Tower, Saint Louis, MO 63119-2408.
E-mail address: meyersb@wustl.edu

Surg Clin N Am 90 (2010) 935–953
doi:10.1016/j.suc.2010.06.008
0039-6109/10/$ – see front matter © 2010 Published by Elsevier Inc.

surgical.theclinics.com

usually caused by rupture of apical subpleural blebs in otherwise normal lungs. The reported incidence varies from 7.4 per 100,000 per year in the United States to 24 per 100,000 per year in the United Kingdom. The incidence in women is lower: 1.2 per 1000,000 per year in the United States and 9.8 per 100,000 per year in the United Kingdom.[1–4] In the United States, primary spontaneous pneumothoraces affect more than 20,000 patients per year and may account for as much as $130,000,000 in health care expenditures annually.[2,5] Compared with nonsmokers, the relative risk of pneumothorax in smokers is 22 times greater for men and 9 times greater for women.[6]

When a spontaneous pneumothorax occurs in patients with known underlying lung disease, it is referred to as secondary spontaneous pneumothorax. Causes include bullous diseases (chronic obstructive pulmonary disease [COPD] and emphysema), cystic diseases (cystic fibrosis, lymphangioleiomyomatosis), infectious causes (pneumonia, severe acute respiratory syndrome), catamenial, connective tissue disorders (Marfan syndrome), and malignancy (primary lung cancer, metastatic disease). The incidence of secondary spontaneous pneumothorax in the United States is 6.3 per 1000,000 per year in men and 2 per 100,000 per year in women.[2] Most of these cases are caused by hyperinflation and rupture of bullae.

Traumatic pneumothoraces can result from both blunt and penetrating injuries to the chest wall, bronchi, lung, or esophagus. Iatrogenic pneumothoraces can occur after diagnostic or therapeutic interventions.

Patient Presentation

Patients who develop a pneumothorax usually complain of sudden onset of dyspnea and pleuritic chest pain. However, the condition may be asymptomatic in 10% of cases. Forty-six percent of patients with primary pneumothorax wait more than 2 days after onset of symptoms before seeing a physician.[4] Patients with secondary spontaneous pneumothorax may have more severe symptoms because they have less pulmonary reserve because of their underlying lung disease. On physical examination, patients typically have decreased breath sounds, decreased chest excursions, and hyperresonant percussion on the affected side. Subcutaneous emphysema may also be present. If the patient has any hemodynamic instability, the concern for a tension pneumothorax must be raised. Additional signs of a tension pneumothorax include significant respiratory distress, tachypnea, distended neck veins, pulsus paradoxus, displacement of the point of maximal cardiac impulse, and trachea shift. These signs are often late and emergency treatment must be initiated with an urgent thoracostomy tube or temporary decompression of the chest with a 14- to 16-gauge needle or catheter placed in the second intercostal space in the midclavicular line on the affected side.

Clinical Findings

Chest radiographs can show the pneumothorax as a hyperlucent area with an absence of pulmonary markings. A white visceral pleural line can be seen outlining the collapsed lung border (**Fig. 1**). Lateral displacement of the mediastinum and/or trachea and downward displacement of the diaphragm can be seen with a tension pneumothorax. According to the British Thoracic Society guidelines, a pneumothorax is defined as small if the distance from the chest wall to the visceral pleural line is less than 2 cm, or large if the distance is greater than 2 cm.[4] However, the American College of Chest Physicians defines small pneumothoraces as those in which the visceral pleura is less than 3 cm from the chest wall and large pneumothoraces as those more than 3 cm.[3] The chest cavity is a three-dimensional space and it is difficult to accurately calculate the size of the pneumothorax using plain chest films. It has

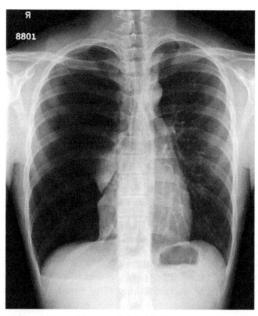

Fig. 1. Twenty-year-old man with a right-sided spontaneous pneumothorax. The compressed and collapsed right lung, and the widened intercostal distance on the right side, all suggest a degree of tension pneumothorax is present. Successful management took place with a 19 French percutaneous chest catheter.

been estimated that, if the pneumothorax is 1 cm wide, it accounts for 25% of the hemithorax volume. A 2-cm pneumothorax can occupy up to 50% of the chest cavity. In patients with COPD, a large apical bulla can be misdiagnosed as a pneumothorax because of a similar appearance on chest radiograph. Chest computed tomography (CT) can help differentiate between these two conditions and provide information on underlying lung pathology. A large left-sided pneumothorax may lead to a right-sided shift in the QRS axis on an electrocardiogram, with a decrease in the precordial R wave voltage. In general, once the pneumothorax is treated, the electrocardiogram reading will return to normal.[7]

Nonoperative Management

There are 3 principles for treatment of a pneumothorax: (1) eliminate the intrapleural air collection, (2) facilitate pleural healing, and (3) prevent recurrence. Initial treatment options include one or more of the following options: observation, supplemental oxygen, needle aspiration of intrapleural air, chest tube insertion, and thoracoscopic or thoracotomy interventions. The patient's clinical status is the most important factor to consider in proper management.

An asymptomatic patient in good health with a small (less than 2 cm) pneumothorax can be managed expectantly with observation. Spontaneous reabsorption of pneumothoraces has been estimated at 1.25% to 1.8% (about 50–70 mL) of the total volume of air in the pleural space per day.[8] The administration of supplemental oxygen reduces the partial pressure of nitrogen in the pleural capillaries and increases air reabsorption from the pleural space.[4,9] If patients are treated expectantly with observation, it is important to follow them closely with serial chest radiographs to make sure the pneumothorax is resolving. With observation, a 25% pneumothorax can take as long as 20 days to reabsorb.

In patients with mild to moderate respiratory symptoms and a moderate or large first-time pneumothorax, a trial of needle aspiration should be considered. Two recent randomized controlled studies have been conducted evaluating needle aspiration versus chest tube insertion. One study consisted of 60 participants with either a first episode of primary spontaneous pneumothorax, or a pneumothorax greater than 20%. The patients were randomized into one of 2 treatment groups: manual pleural aspiration with a small-caliber 16-gauge intravenous catheter under local anesthesia, or chest tube drainage with a 16 to 20 French chest tube. Patients with underlying lung disease, previous pneumothorax, or tension pneumothorax were excluded from the study. The results showed no difference in the immediate success rate, early failure rate, 1-year success rate, or complication rate of simple aspiration versus intercostal tube drainage. Simple aspiration had an immediate success rate of 60%, and resulted in a significant reduction in the proportion of patients hospitalized compared with intercostal tube drainage.[10]

The second study enrolled 137 patients with a first episode of primary spontaneous pneumothorax at a single center. Patients were included if they were symptomatic or had greater than a 20% pneumothorax. Once again, patients were randomized to simple aspiration versus tube thoracostomy. The results showed no difference in immediate success rate, 1-week success rate, complication rate, recurrence at 3-month follow-up, or recurrence at 1 and 2 years. Only 26% of the patients treated with simple aspiration required hospital admission, versus 100% of those receiving chest tubes.[11] A Cochrane Review of this topic concurred with the British Thoracic Surgery guidelines recommending simple aspiration as a first-line treatment of primary spontaneous pneumothoraces requiring intervention.[4,12]

Conventional tube thoracostomy should be used in patients with large pneumothoraces who fail needle aspiration, who have underlying lung pathology, or who are very symptomatic. Chest tubes are inserted in the anterior or midaxillary line in the fourth or fifth interspace and should be guided posteriorly and cephalad. This tube positioning allows drainage of both fluid and air. If the patient has an isolated pneumothorax with no pleural effusion, a small chest tube (16–20 French) can be used to minimize discomfort to the patient. With proper tube drainage, the lung should re-expand rapidly. Negative pressure (-10 to -20 cm H_2O) on the chest tube or underwater seal can be used to maintain lung re-expansion. The chest tube can be removed after the air leak has stopped. If the air leak is prolonged and the patient can maintain full lung expansion on underwater seal drainage, a 1-way valve can be placed at the end of the tube and the patient discharged and followed as an outpatient.

Surgical Treatment

Most cases of primary spontaneous pneumothorax resolve with nonoperative management; however, some require surgical intervention. The indications for operative intervention include persistent air leak, failure of the lung to fully expand with chest tube drainage, hemothorax, recurrent pneumothorax, bilateral pneumothorax, first occurrence of contralateral pneumothorax, high-risk activities/professions, and poor access to medical treatment or follow-up.

Most air leaks seal within 48 hours after placement of a chest tube, but up to 5% have a prolonged air leak lasting more than 4 days.[13] Recurrence rates vary widely depending on the treatment applied and the follow-up period. In general, recurrence rates of primary pneumothorax range from 16% to 52% with follow-up of 10 years.

Recurrence rates for secondary pneumothorax range from 40% to 56%.[14–16] Recurrence most often occurred within 6 months following the first episode. Sadikot and colleagues[17] followed 154 patients with primary pneumothorax for 54 months and observed a recurrence rate of 39% within the first year.

Patients who are involved in professions or recreations that involve rapid changes in atmospheric pressure, such as scuba divers or airline personnel, should have their pneumothoraces treated surgically at initial presentation, given their increased risk should they have a recurrence. The British Thoracic Society recommends that patients with a pneumothorax should not fly for 72 hours after a pleural drainage tube is removed, and only then if a chest radiograph at 48 hours after tube removal confirms resolution of the pneumothorax.[4] Patients with limited access to medical services should be offered surgical treatment because of the dangers of developing a recurrent pneumothorax and not being able to get it treated in a timely fashion.

The principles of surgical intervention are to resect any blebs or bullae and to obliterate the pleural space to avoid recurrences. Chest CT scans can help delineate the surgical anatomy. For patients with a primary spontaneous pneumothorax, 30% to 40% of patients have single or multiple blebs. These blebs are often found at the apex of the upper lobe or the superior segment of the lower lobe. An additional 5% to 10% of patients have bullae that are larger than 2 cm. However, 12% to 15% of patients have normal lung with adhesions suggesting previous pneumothoraces. Between 30% and 40% have no obvious pathologic explanation for their pneumothorax and normal lungs.

Resection of blebs with stapling has been shown to decrease the recurrence rate from 23% to 1.8%. Even if no abnormalities were found in the lung, resection of the apex decreased the recurrence rate.[18] It is important to combine a resection with a technique that locally fuses the pleural space to reduce the recurrence rate. This fusion can be achieved by pleurectomy, pleural abrasion, or pleurodesis. All these methods create an inflammatory reaction causing the lung to adhere to the chest wall, thus precluding collapse of the lung in the event of another parenchymal air leak. Thus, the procedure does not prevent an air leak from occurring; instead it is aimed at preventing a significant pneumothorax from developing. When used alone, the recurrence rate after pleurectomy is 1% to 5%.[19] Pleural abrasion is technically easier and is associated with fewer hemorrhagic complications than pleurectomy. In a review of 9 case series, the recurrence rate of pneumothorax after pleural abrasion alone was 2.3%.[20] Chemical pleurodesis can be used at the time of surgery, or via a chest tube in patients who are not candidates for surgical intervention. Talc is most often used for chemical pleurodesis, but autologous blood, bleomycin, tetracycline, and doxycycline have all been used.[21,22] Talc is a powder of hydrous magnesium silicate and is extremely effective in inducing pleural adhesions. Talc pleurodesis is effective, with recurrence rates of 5% to 8% when patients are treated with talc pleurodesis alone.[23,24] However, it induces fever and pain and, in up to 2% of patients, the associated pneumonitis can induce respiratory failure.[25] In addition, there is concern about the long-term consequences of leaving foreign material (talc crystals) in the chest cavity in young patients. Intrapleural injection of tetracycline alone is less effective and has been associated with recurrence rates of 16%.[26] Injection of tetracycline or doxycycline can be painful and it is important to premedicate patients with analgesics. Intrapleural lidocaine injection can be added to help with analgesia.

Traditionally, a posterolateral or transaxillary thoracotomy was used for the surgical approach. However, the development of video-assisted thoracoscopic surgery (VATS) has greatly decreased the morbidity associated with the surgical treatment of pneumothoraces. VATS provides excellent visualization and is associated with decreased pain and length of hospital stay. With VATS, an endoscopic stapler can be used to resect diseased lung tissue, and a pleurectomy, pleural abrasion, and chemical pleurodesis can be performed at the same time. In a prospective, controlled, randomized study of 60 patients with spontaneous pneumothorax who were treated with either VATS or posterolateral thoracotomy, VATS was associated with decreased analgesic requirement and a shorter hospitalization. There were no significant differences between operative failures, duration of chest tube drainage, treatment failures, or recurrences with the two approaches.[27] A systematic review of the literature comparing VATS with traditional surgical approaches also found decreased use of pain medication and shorter hospital stay in the patients having VATS.[28] Whenever possible, a VATS approach should be used to treat pneumothoraces when surgical intervention is indicated.

Pneumothorax Summary

Pneumothoraces are among the more common problems that the thoracic surgeon is asked to manage. Most primary pneumothoraces can be managed with minimal, if any, intervention. For more complicated patients, a surgical bleb resection with pleurodesis provides reproducibly good results. Similar results can be obtained via VATS, with shorter hospital stays and less pain for the patient.

BULLOUS DISEASE
Definition

A bulla is defined as an air-filled space, 1 cm or more in distended diameter, that forms within the lung parenchyma, typically as a result of emphysematous destruction. Anatomically, bullae have a thin outer wall consisting of the visceral pleura and an inner wall consisting of the remnants of emphysematous lung. The inside of the bullae can be either smooth or crossed with fibrous bands, which are likely the remnants of alveolar and interlobular septa.[29] Multiple dilated, thin-walled vessels can pass through the walls of bullae, or be suspended within the fibrous septa. Rarely, bullae may enlarge to a degree that they occupy more than one-third of the hemithorax; in this circumstance, the term giant bulla is applied.

Patients with bullae have traditionally been divided into 2 groups: those in whom the remaining lung parenchyma is structurally normal, and those in whom the rest of the lung exhibits emphysematous change. The latter group can be described as having bullous emphysema. There have been several proposed classification systems for giant bullae, based on the number, shape, and position of the bullae, combined with the condition of the underlying lung.[30–32] Although such classification systems are potentially useful, the lack of widespread usage limits their clinical usefulness.

Natural History of Bullae

In 1968, Boushy reported on 49 patients with bullous emphysema who were followed with serial chest radiographs and pulmonary function tests.[33] Of the 49 patients reported, 27 had giant bullae. The investigators noted a consistent tendency toward growth of the bullae over time, with concomitant worsening pulmonary function. Some of these patients had a gradual worsening, whereas some were stable for several years before worsening. There were 4 notable patients whose bullae decreased in size; in all 4, the bullae had become infected. Although giant bullae may be asymptomatic on presentation, they typically do not remain so.[34] There have been some case reports of bullae regressing,[35–37] but the natural history of bullae seems to show a pattern of progressive, if unpredictable, enlargement.

Evaluation and Decision Making

Initial investigation is directed toward identifying patients who are most likely to benefit from resection of bullae. This investigation includes an evaluation of the overall medical status of the patient for the assessment of any major comorbidities that would preclude a resection. The patient's cardiac status is considered for the presence of cor pulmonale, right-sided heart failure, as well as for risk stratification for other perioperative cardiac events. For operative planning, and determination of operability, pulmonary function tests and a CT scan of the chest are usually sufficient.

Pulmonary function testing

In patients with a localized giant bulla and normal-appearing underlying lung, FitzGerald and colleagues[38] showed a strong correlation between the patient's decline in forced expiratory volume in the first second of expiration (FEV_1), the size of the bulla, and the improvement in postoperative FEV_1. In an additional longitudinal study, Ohta and colleagues[39] followed 25 patients having bullectomy for 4 years. They identified 20 patients with durable improvement in symptoms, and 5 patients whose symptoms worsened after 1 year. Only a higher initial FEV_1 and a uniform distribution of ventilation were able to predict the sustained postoperative improvement.[39]

It is difficult to determine whether a patient's reduced FEV_1 is secondary to the presence of the bulla or to the emphysema in the underlying lung. This distinction is important, because performing a giant bullectomy on a patient with substantial underlying emphysema has been associated with higher morbidity and mortality,[40,41] as well as less-durable benefit.[38] Using CT lung density measurements, Gould and colleagues[42] found that pulmonary function testing correlates poorly with the degree of bullous change, but is strongly related to the degree of emphysema in the underlying lung. Haerens and colleagues[43] reported on 15 patients having bullectomy, 10 of whom had generalized emphysema and 5 who had normal underlying lung. Preoperatively, the FEV_1 of the patients with normal underlying lung was higher, but, on an individual patient basis, it was impossible to predict the quality of the underlying lung based solely on pulmonary function testing.[43]

A reduction in diffusion capacity of carbon monoxide in the lung (DLCO) has been noted as an indicator of underlying emphysema,[44,45] and patients with normal DLCO have been found to have better short- and long- term outcomes after bullae resection.[38,46,47] However, reversible conditions leading to extreme airway obstruction can give falsely depressed DLCO levels; as such, a low DLCO should not be the sole reason for denying a patient an operation.

There is no generally accepted absolute cutoff in pulmonary function values for which surgery is contraindicated. Even with an extremely low FEV_1, patients with preserved underlying lung tissue can obtain substantial improvement in both symptoms and pulmonary function after resection of giant bullae.[38,48] The determination of the nature of the underlying lung function is best obtained by CT scan.

Chest CT

CT provides valuable information about the architecture of the diseased lung parenchyma, and should be obtained for all patients being considered for bullectomy.[49,50] The size, location, and number of bullae can be well visualized, in addition to any other abnormalities such as masses or infiltrates. The consistency of the underlying lung can also be assessed (**Fig. 2**). Morgan and colleagues[49] used CT to evaluate 43 patients

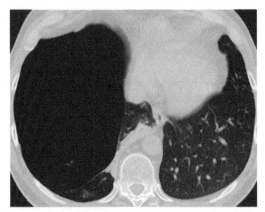

Fig. 2. Several different states of lung disease present in a patient with giant bulla. The large right-sided bulla is evident as the homogeneous hypodense region in the right hemi-thorax. Some residual septae are evident posteriorly and medially. There is comparatively normal lung on the opposite side. There is compressed and atelectatic lung adjacent to the mediastinum, likely caused by the pressure of the bulla.

with apparent bullous disease. CT differentiated 20 patients whose bullae were merely local exaggerations of generalized emphysema from 23 patients who had well-defined bullae with relatively normal underlying lung. There was no statistical difference in the pulmonary function tests between these groups.

Indications for Operation

In 1950, Baldwin and colleagues[51] suggested that ventilatory insufficiency and the absence of generalized emphysema were the criteria predicting the need for, and success of, bullectomy. Sixty years later, the standard criteria have not significantly changed: isolated bullae occupying more than 30% of the hemothorax, the preservation of underlying lung parenchyma, and a patient who has dyspnea.

Although the first 2 criteria are best evaluated via chest CT, the presence of symptoms is subjective. Dyspnea can be measured using either the modified Hugh-Jones Criteria[52] or the Medical Research Council Dyspnea Scale[53]; any grade of dyspnea greater than zero on either scale is abnormal, and is considered symptomatic. For those symptomatic patients with a giant bullae and otherwise preserved lung function, there is little argument that they will benefit from surgical treatment. Patients with severe underlying emphysema are best considered in the context of lung volume reduction surgery (LVRS). Other, more controversial, indications include bullae in an asymptomatic patient, hemoptysis, and chest pain.

Asymptomatic patient

The natural history of bullous disease is progressive enlargement of the bullae, with concomitant worsening of pulmonary function. Some have advocated that surgery is indicated in the absence of symptoms, provided a giant bulla occupies more than 50% of the hemithorax, the adjacent lung is compressed, or the bulla has enlarged during a period of years.[54,55] Others think that the incidence of postoperative complications is too high to justify operating on an asymptomatic patient.[34,40,56]

Hemoptysis

Massive hemoptysis has rarely been associated with rupture of vessels in a giant bulla.[57] In their extended series, Gaensler and colleagues[46] noted only 1 bullectomy that was performed because of bleeding. Because of the rarity of hemoptysis solely explicable by bullous disease, hemoptysis in this patient population mandates an investigation for other potential sources, such as carcinoma, bronchiectasis, or aspergillus superinfection.[29]

Chest pain

Chest pain associated with giant bullae has been reported. It can be substernal, radiating to the arms, and exercise related. It is hypothesized to be secondary to air trapping in a bulla, with subsequent distention of the visceral or mediastinal parietal pleura. Once cardiac causes have been eliminated, surgical treatment of bullae has been performed for chest pain with good results.[46]

Surgical Approaches

Open bullectomy

The goal of bullectomy is to resect as much bullous disease as possible while minimizing resection of the spared lung. Care is taken in opening the pleural space, because injury to the underlying parenchyma can be difficult to repair, and the resulting air leak can be prolonged. A complete adhesiolysis reveals the full extent of the bullous disease, and allows the underlying lung to fully expand. Unless an operation for cancer is being performed, anatomic resections are generally unnecessary.[48] Once the bullae are clearly identified, there are several acceptable approaches.

This first open approach, perhaps of historical interest at best, involves using the wall of the bulla to buttress a staple line across the base of the bulla. The largest bulla is opened longitudinally, and its cavity is explored from within, dividing any septa. Allis clamps are used to grasp the bulla from the inside at the reflection of the bullous wall with normal lung; this interface can be identified by gently ventilating the operative lung. The wall of the bulla is folded over and used as a staple line buttress, and a linear stapler is fired completely across the base of the bulla. At completion, all raw surfaces are sealed, and the buttressed staple line consists of 4 layers of parietal pleura and bulla wall.[58]

Alternatively, a giant bulla can be excised without widely opening the bulla. The bulla is deflated by making a small incision the lateral wall, which is grasped and held up with Allis clamps, and sequential firings of a linear stapler are applied.[59–62] Compression of the area of the lung where the stapler is to be applied, with either the surgeon's fingers or a straight clamp, can ease the application of the stapler and prevent injury to the underlying lung. Again, emphasis is placed on leaving behind as much normal underlying parenchyma as possible.

Bullae may also be removed by simple excision with suturing of any air leaks. The wall of the bulla is excised down to the interface with normal lung, and any visualized air leaks at the base of the bulla are sutured closed.[63] This technique is not commonly used in modern practice.

Both thoracotomy and median sternotomy have been used as approaches for open bullectomy, without a clear advantage being shown for either approach. For patients with bilateral disease, a median sternotomy provides access to both pleural spaces, and, as such, is the preferred approach in these cases.[43] However, patients with bilateral giant bullae and preserved underlying lung function are rare, and finding such a case should raise the suspicion of more severe emphysema in the underlying lung.

Thoracoscopic bullectomy

Because thoracoscopy has the advantage of avoiding the pain and disability of a thoracotomy, many surgeons have adopted thoracoscopy for the treatment of giant bullae. Wakabayashi[64] reported the first series of thoracoscopically treated giant bullae in 1993. Both bilateral and unilateral thoracoscopic-stapled bullectomy procedures have been performed. As with open bullectomy, care must be taken when entering the pleura to avoid injuring the underlying lung, and a complete adhesiolysis is needed to visualize the bulla to be resected. The bulla can be partially opened to obtain adequate visualization. Once the bulla is identified, a stapled bullectomy can be performed with sequential firings of a buttressed endoscopic stapler, in a manner similar to the open bullectomy.[59–62] The underlying lung is reinflated under direct vision; if the underlying lung does not reinflate, bronchoscopy should be performed to suction clean the involved airways. When there has been chronic collapse of a section of lung, it can sometimes be difficult to re-expand. Typically, the airway pressure necessary to inflate the collapsed segment is high and, as a consequence, the abnormally compliant diseased lung is preferentially inflated. If this occurs, it can be useful to pass a small catheter through the working port of the bronchoscope and apply gentle jet ventilation to the airway leading to the collapsed lung segment.

Although the presence of a previous thoracotomy is a relative contraindication to subsequent thoracoscopic procedures, there have been successful series of patients in whom thoracoscopic bullectomy was performed despite previous thoracotomy.[65]

Endocavitary drainage

Monaldi originally described a technique for endocavitary drainage of tuberculous cavities in 1938,[66] and this technique was adapted for giant bullae in 1995.[67] In this technique, a small thoracotomy is made over the site of the bulla. A segment of rib is resected, and the parietal pleura adjacent to the bulla is incised. An incision is made on the lateral wall of the bulla, and any septae in the interior of the bulla are excised. Two purse-string sutures are placed around the hole in the bulla, and a 32 French Foley catheter is inserted into the bulla to serve as an endocavitary drain. The balloon on the Foley is inflated, the purse-string sutures are tied, and suction is applied to the Foley, collapsing the bulla. The pleural drain is discontinued after 48 hours, whereas the endocavitary drain is removed in 8 to 21 days.[67,68]

Endocavitary drainage of giant bullae offers a limited surgical approach that avoids resection of underlying lung while providing symptomatic relief and functional improvement. Most investigators reserve this treatment for patients who would not otherwise tolerate a thoracotomy,[68] but some advocate it as the first surgical choice for any patient with a giant bullae.[69]

Surgical Outcomes

Symptomatic improvement has been reported in 80% to 100% of postoperative patients in numerous studies.[39,70–74] Many studies have also shown postoperative improvement in pulmonary function, although there is a wide range (24%–200%) in the degree of improvement in FEV_1, for example.[38,73,75] Limited long-term data suggest that the postoperative increase in lung function tends to degrade with time, with the loss of function related to the condition of the underlying lung.[38]

Operative mortality is low, ranging from 0% to 5% in several studies.[38,73–75] In contrast, operative morbidity is substantial, with most postoperative complications involving a prolonged air leak. The frequency of prolonged air leak is approximately 50% in most series.[73,75]

Several studies have been performed to try to minimize the incidence and length of air leaks. Gentle handling of the lung tissue remains of paramount importance. The use of buttressed staple lines and surgical sealants has failed to show effectiveness in pulmonary resections as a whole.[60,76–78] In contrast, there is evidence that, in the particular subset of patients with emphysematous lung, the use of buttresses[59,61] and sealants[79] can decrease both the duration and severity of air leaks. Early placement of the pleural drains to water seal, rather than suction, has been shown to assist with sealing of air leaks.[80]

Summary

The best candidates for surgical resection of giant bullae are patients with an isolated bulla occupying more than 30% of the hemithorax, collapsed but otherwise normal underlying lung, and dyspnea. Several operative techniques have been used to accomplish these goals, including stapled bullectomy, excision, ligation, and endocavitary drainage. In properly selected patients, most can be expected to have subjective improvement of their dyspnea as well as demonstrable improvement in pulmonary function testing. The long-term persistence of this improvement is dependent on the quality of the underlying lung and the progression of any disease in that lung.

Emphysema

In 1993, Cooper observed that patients with COPD, in the process of undergoing a lung transplant, were able to get adequate gas exchange from an emphysematous lung if properly ventilated.[81] In addition, transplanting normal-sized lungs into a hyperexpanded chest led to restoration of a normal thoracic cavity. These observations led Cooper to resurrect the idea of lung volume reduction, with some modifications of an approach described 40 years earlier by Brantigan.[81] The procedure was considered palliative, intended to reduce dyspnea and increase exercise tolerance, and able to achieve these goals in carefully selected patients.

Following this sentinel report, LVRS enjoyed widespread application within the United States. However, analysis of patients undergoing this procedure revealed an unacceptably high mortality: 23% at 12 months.[82] This led to cessation of federal funding for the operation, and a decrease in enthusiasm for the procedure. To more rigorously evaluate the benefit of the operation, the National Institute of Health sponsored a large, multicenter trial that began enrolling patients in 1999.[83] The trial, called the National Emphysema Treatment Trial (NETT), was a prospective randomized study of 1218 patients, and it has provided strong evidence for the efficacy, safety, and durability of LVRS. The outcomes from the NETT analysis, in conjunction with data from earlier trials, help provide the criteria for defining which patients will benefit from LVRS.

Patient Selection

The goals of preoperative assessment for LVRS are to identify patients who remain disabled by emphysema despite maximal medical therapy, determine which patients will benefit from surgery with an acceptable risk, and exclude those patients with an increased risk of poor outcome.

Medical management and preparation

The first step is to assess the patient's symptoms and degree of quality-of-life impairment related to emphysema. Patients with severe, incapacitating emphysema are considered for surgical intervention. A structured pulmonary rehabilitation program is a critical first step in determining suitability for an operation. The program should include abstinence from tobacco products, an exercise training program, optimization of medical treatment, patient education, and psychosocial assessment. Exercise training is designed to increase endurance and decrease exertional dyspnea. Patients enrolled at the authors' LVRS program are required to complete an exercise program that has a goal of 30 minutes of daily continuous exercise, 5 days a week, on a treadmill or stationary bicycle. The Joint Commission on Accreditation of Hospitals and Organizations also uses a minimal performance of 3 minutes of unloaded pedaling on a stationary bicycle as a prerequisite for LVRS surgery in the United States. A significant number of patients achieve enough improvement in their symptoms that they decline LVRS after undergoing exercise-based pulmonary rehabilitation.[84,85] Exercise tolerance also has an important postoperative predictive value: the NETT trial demonstrated that, in patients with upper lobe predominant disease, patients with high exercise tolerance (ie, less impaired by the disease) did not have the same survival benefit from surgery as those more impaired patients with low exercise tolerance.[86] However, other clinical trials have amended enrollment criteria after observing an excessive mortality in the patients with the poorest exercise abilities. It is clear that patients selected for surgical therapy must be impaired enough to merit the risks of surgery, but not so ill that they cannot participate in physical therapy.

Medical optimization includes several factors. Oxygen therapy is indicated for any patient with a Pao_2 less that 55 mm Hg, or an Sao_2 less than 88%. Bronchodilator therapy is useful for alleviating symptomatic airflow limitation; however, many patients use appropriately prescribed inhalers incorrectly. Assuring the correct use of inhalers should be a component of any medical evaluation. Many patients with stable COPD symptoms use long-term corticosteroid therapy, despite the absence of prospective data supporting a benefit of steroids on lung function or its rate of decline. As such, tapering the use of corticosteroids preoperatively to the lowest possible dose is advised in an effort to avoid the associated risks of poor wound healing and infection.

Cardiovascular function

As with any other major operation, assessment of cardiac function is a critical component of an evaluation for emphysema surgery. Rest and stress echocardiography, radionuclide ventriculograms, thallium imaging, and other studies can assist with cardiac risk stratification. However, the patient with COPD provides several unique challenges to these modalities, limiting the usefulness of such tests. Exercise testing is rarely useful because of the patient's inability to exercise to maximal heart rates. Chest hyperinflation can limit the visualization afforded by echocardiography, and concerns about bronchoconstriction may limit the use of dipyridimole or adenosine. As such, many otherwise acceptable surgical candidates eventually undergo right and left heart catheterization just before surgery. Any intervention must be coordinated among all physicians involved, because the placement of a drug-eluting coronary stent in a preoperative patient can have major implications on the timing and the conduct of the surgery.

Pulmonary function

Spirometry is the cornerstone of pulmonary function testing, because it provides quantifiable, reproducible assessment of several aspects of pulmonary physiology. Airflow obstruction is the most significant abnormality with emphysema; it can be accurately estimated by forced expiratory maneuvers. Lung volumes, measured by plethysmography, indicate the degree of trapped gas and residual volume. Resting and exercise arterial blood gas analyses indicate the patient's pulmonary reserve, and reflect their potential for recovery after surgery. Diffusing capacity, as measured by DLCO values, estimates the severity of the disease within the pulmonary vascular bed. These parameters provide objective criteria for assessment of emphysema severity, and serve as markers of the patients at highest risk of a poor outcome.

Radiographic evaluation

The purpose of imaging preoperative patients is to identify those patients with findings favorable for surgical intervention. The main features to assess are the presence of hyperinflation, the severity of emphysema, and the distribution of emphysema.

The severity and distribution of emphysema correlates with clinical outcomes after surgery. The greatest improvements in FEV_1 and exercise capacity tend to occur in patients with more-severe, heterogeneous disease that predominates in the upper lobes (**Fig. 3**A, B).[87,88] The standard chest CT examination is the most accurate means of evaluating the severity and distribution of emphysema. However, there is

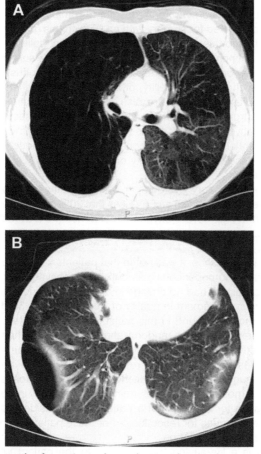

Fig. 3. (A) CT radiograph of a patient who underwent lung reduction surgery. Both upper lobes are diseased. The right side shows more extensive bullous changes, whereas the left side has emphysematous destruction without macroscopic bullae. (B) Lower cuts in the same the patient show relatively normal lung parenchyma and pulmonary vessels near the base of the lungs. This degree of heterogeneity is often seen in the patients who experience the best response to LVRS.

considerable variation in the interpretation of CT scans in these patients; the entire lung is affected to some degree by emphysema, and it may be difficult to assess the heterogeneity of the disease. Studies have found considerable interobserver variability in interpretation of the distribution of emphysema on CT.[89] Despite this, CT remains the mainstay of preoperative imaging.

Nuclear medicine ventilation-perfusion lung scans depicting regional blood flow patterns provide a valuable roadmap for surgery. As the distribution of the perfusion agent is relative, the absolute severity of emphysema cannot be assessed, but the presence of diffuse versus upper or lower lobe predominant disease can be identified. In addition, a right- or left-sided predominance of lung function may direct surgery toward a unilateral approach, if the findings are also supported by the CT.

LVRS versus Transplantation

Given the potential morbidity associated with surgical intervention, it is worth re-emphasizing that these procedure should only be considered for patients who continue to have debilitating symptoms despite maximal medical therapy. It is rare that patients are considered for surgery with an FEV_1 that is greater than 40% of predicted. The exception to this would be a patient with giant bulla as described earlier.

Similarly, significant nonpulmonary comorbidities eliminate surgery as an option for the patient. These comorbidities include extremes of body habitus, concurrent malignant processes, psychosocial instability, or advanced age. Patients who have used tobacco within the last 6 months are also excluded from surgical consideration. Previous thoracic surgical interventions, such as a wedge resection, lobectomy, or pleurodesis, are relative contraindications to ipsilateral bullectomy or LVRS, although contralateral interventions are viable options. In contrast, although previous thoracic operations increase the technical difficulty of the explant, they are not contraindications to transplantation.

With progressive pulmonary dysfunction, the morbidity and mortality associated with LVRS increases. Patients with an FEV_1 less that 20% of predicted, marked hypercarbia ($Pa_{CO_2} > 55$ mm Hg), severe oxygen dependence (>6 L at rest), or with pulmonary hypertension, are all relative indicators that the patient may be better served by transplantation than LVRS.

Early in the NETT experience, it was noted that patients with an FEV_1 less than 20% of predicted and either homogeneous distribution of emphysema on CT or a DLCO of less than 20% of predicted had no change in exercise tolerance, no improvement in FEV_1, no subjective improvement in quality of life, and a 16% 30-day mortality after LVRS.[90] The high mortality found in this patient cohort prompted a modification of the NETT protocol, excluding from randomization any patients who met these criteria. However, retrospective review of a patient population that met the high-risk criteria of the NETT protocol showed improved respiratory function at an acceptable risk of mortality.[91] This suggests that the presence of suitable anatomic heterogeneity of disease may be the most important determinant of outcome. In our experience, the most common reason for exclusion of a patient from consideration of LVRS is the lack of sufficient target areas for resection.[92] For these patients, lung transplantation is the only remaining surgical option.

Lung transplant is a life-saving tool available to the patient who is critically ill; patients with severe physiologic derangements and unfavorable disease anatomy have dramatic initial improvements after transplant.[93] In patients who would qualify for both transplant and LVRS, it is tempting to consider listing the patient for transplant. However, despite the improvements that have been made in lung transplants in the last 20 years, mortality remains approximately 50% at 5 years.[94]

SUMMARY

Surgical intervention is a viable option in a select group of patients with severe, incapacitating emphysema. Only those patients who have failed to progress despite optimized medical therapy and a rigorous pulmonary rehabilitation regimen should be considered for surgical intervention. Pulmonary function tests, CT, and nuclear ventilation-perfusion scans further delineate those patients who are most likely to benefit from the operation, as well as determining which intervention is most likely to have a good outcome. The surgical options available to the patient depend on the spectrum of the distribution of their disease; isolated bullae can be treated with bullectomy, heterogeneous emphysema lends itself to LVRS, whereas homogeneous disease is best treated by lung transplantation. The ideal indicators for LVRS also include hyperinflation, an FEV_1 greater that 20%, and a normal $Paco_2$. In contrast, patients with a low FEV_1, hypercapnia, and associated pulmonary hypertension are directed toward transplantation.

REFERENCES

1. Gupta D, Hansell A, Nichols T, et al. Epidemiology of pneumothorax in England. Thorax 2000;55(8):666–71.
2. Melton LJ 3rd, Hepper NG, Offord KP. Incidence of spontaneous pneumothorax in Olmsted County, Minnesota: 1950 to 1974. Am Rev Respir Dis 1979;120(6): 1379–82.
3. Baumann MH, Strange C, Heffner JE, et al. Management of spontaneous pneumothorax: an American College of Chest Physicians Delphi consensus statement. Chest 2001;119(2):590–602.
4. Henry M, Arnold T, Harvey J. BTS guidelines for the management of spontaneous pneumothorax. Thorax 2003;58(Suppl 2):ii39–52.
5. Bense L, Wiman LG, Jendteg S, et al. Economic costs of spontaneous pneumothorax. Chest 1991;99(1):260–1.
6. Bense L, Eklund G, Wiman LG. Smoking and the increased risk of contracting spontaneous pneumothorax. Chest 1987;92(6):1009–12.
7. Walston A, Brewer DL, Kitchens CS, et al. The electrocardiographic manifestations of spontaneous left pneumothorax. Ann Intern Med 1974;80(3):375–9.
8. Kircher LT Jr, Swartzel RL. Spontaneous pneumothorax and its treatment. J Am Med Assoc 1954;155(1):24–9.
9. Hill RC, DeCarlo DP Jr, Hill JF, et al. Resolution of experimental pneumothorax in rabbits by oxygen therapy. Ann Thorac Surg 1995;59(4):825–7 [discussion 827–8].
10. Noppen M, Alexander P, Driesen P, et al. Manual aspiration versus chest tube drainage in first episodes of primary spontaneous pneumothorax: a multicenter, prospective, randomized pilot study. Am J Respir Crit Care Med 2002;165(9): 1240–4.
11. Ayed AK, Chandrasekaran C, Sukumar M. Aspiration versus tube drainage in primary spontaneous pneumothorax: a randomised study. Eur Respir J 2006; 27(3):477–82.
12. Wakai A, O'Sullivan RG, McCabe G. Simple aspiration versus intercostal tube drainage for primary spontaneous pneumothorax in adults. Cochrane Database Syst Rev 2007;1:CD004479.
13. Schoenenberger RA, Haefeli WE, Weiss P, et al. Timing of invasive procedures in therapy for primary and secondary spontaneous pneumothorax. Arch Surg 1991; 126(6):764–6.

14. Schramel FM, Postmus PE, Vanderschueren RG. Current aspects of spontaneous pneumothorax. Eur Respir J 1997;10(6):1372–9.
15. Lippert HL, Lund O, Blegvad S, et al. Independent risk factors for cumulative recurrence rate after first spontaneous pneumothorax. Eur Respir J 1991;4(3): 324–31.
16. Videm V, Pillgram-Larsen J, Ellingsen O, et al. Spontaneous pneumothorax in chronic obstructive pulmonary disease: complications, treatment and recurrences. Eur J Respir Dis 1987;71(5):365–71.
17. Sadikot RT, Greene T, Meadows K, et al. Recurrence of primary spontaneous pneumothorax. Thorax 1997;52(9):805–9.
18. Mouroux J, Elkaim D, Padovani B, et al. Video-assisted thoracoscopic treatment of spontaneous pneumothorax: technique and results of one hundred cases. J Thorac Cardiovasc Surg 1996;112(2):385–91.
19. Ferraro P, Beauchamp G, Lord F, et al. Spontaneous primary and secondary pneumothorax: a 10-year study of management alternatives. Can J Surg 1994; 37(3):197–202.
20. Weeden D, Smith GH. Surgical experience in the management of spontaneous pneumothorax, 1972–82. Thorax 1983;38(10):737–43.
21. Robinson CL. Autologous blood for pleurodesis in recurrent and chronic spontaneous pneumothorax. Can J Surg 1987;30(6):428–9.
22. Hnatiuk OW, Dillard TA, Oster CN. Bleomycin sclerotherapy for bilateral pneumothoraces in a patient with AIDS. Ann Intern Med 1990;113(12):988–90.
23. Gyorik S, Erni S, Studler U, et al. Long-term follow-up of thoracoscopic talc pleurodesis for primary spontaneous pneumothorax. Eur Respir J 2007;29(4):757–60.
24. Almind M, Lange P, Viskum K. Spontaneous pneumothorax: comparison of simple drainage, talc pleurodesis, and tetracycline pleurodesis. Thorax 1989; 44(8):627–30.
25. Light RW. Talc should not be used for pleurodesis. Am J Respir Crit Care Med 2000;162(6):2024–6.
26. Olsen PS, Andersen HO. Long-term results after tetracycline pleurodesis in spontaneous pneumothorax. Ann Thorac Surg 1992;53(6):1015–7.
27. Waller DA. Video-assisted thoracoscopic surgery (VATS) in the management of spontaneous pneumothorax. Thorax 1997;52(4):307–8.
28. Sedrakyan A, van der Meulen J, Lewsey J, et al. Video assisted thoracic surgery for treatment of pneumothorax and lung resections: systematic review of randomised clinical trials. BMJ 2004;329(7473):1008.
29. Deslauriers J, Leblanc P. Management of bullous disease. Chest Surg Clin N Am 1994;4(3):539–59.
30. DeVries WC, Wolfe WG. The management of spontaneous pneumothorax and bullous emphysema. Surg Clin North Am 1980;60(4):851–66.
31. Mehran RJ, Deslauriers J. Indications for surgery and patient work-up for bullectomy. Chest Surg Clin N Am 1995;5(4):717–34.
32. Reid L. The Pathology Of Emphysema. London: Lloyd-Luke (Medical Books) Ltd; 1967.
33. Boushy SF, Kohen R, Billig DM, et al. Bullous emphysema: clinical, roentgenologic and physiologic study of 49 patients. Dis Chest 1968;54(4):327–34.
34. Ribet ME. Cystic and bullous lung disease. Ann Thorac Surg 1992;53(6):1147.
35. Rothstein E. Infected emphysematous bullae; report of five cases. Am Rev Tuberc 1954;69(2):287–96.
36. Satoh H, Suyama T, Yamashita YT, et al. Spontaneous regression of multiple emphysematous bullae. Can Respir J 1999;6(5):458–60.

37. Park HY, Lim SY, Park HK, et al. Regression of giant bullous emphysema. Intern Med 2010;49(1):55–7.
38. FitzGerald MX, Keelan PJ, Cugell DW, et al. Long-term results of surgery for bullous emphysema. J Thorac Cardiovasc Surg 1974;68(4):566–87.
39. Ohta M, Nakahara K, Yasumitsu T, et al. Prediction of postoperative performance status in patients with giant bulla. Chest 1992;101(3):668–73.
40. Gunstensen J, McCormack RJ. The surgical management of bullous emphysema. J Thorac Cardiovasc Surg 1973;65(6):920–5.
41. Nakahara K, Nakaoka K, Ohno K, et al. Functional indications for bullectomy of giant bulla. Ann Thorac Surg 1983;35(5):480–7.
42. Gould GA, Redpath AT, Ryan M, et al. Parenchymal emphysema measured by CT lung density correlates with lung function in patients with bullous disease. Eur Respir J 1993;6(5):698–704.
43. Haerens M, Deneffe G, Billiet L, et al. Effect on pulmonary function of surgical treatment of bullous lung disease. Acta Clin Belg 1988;43(5):362–73.
44. Hugh-Jones P, Whimster W. The etiology and management of disabling emphysema. Am Rev Respir Dis 1978;117(2):343–78.
45. Pride NB, Barter CE, Hugh-Jones P. The ventilation of bullae and the effect of their removal on thoracic gas volumes and tests of over-all pulmonary function. Am Rev Respir Dis 1973;107(1):83–98.
46. Gaensler EA, Jederlinic PJ, FitzGerald MX. Patient work-up for bullectomy. J Thorac Imaging 1986;1(2):75–93.
47. Wex P, Ebner H, Dragojevic D. Functional surgery of bullous emphysema. Thorac Cardiovasc Surg 1983;31(6):346–51.
48. Potgieter PD, Benatar SR, Hewitson RP, et al. Surgical treatment of bullous lung disease. Thorax 1981;36(12):885–90.
49. Morgan MD, Denison DM, Strickland B. Value of computed tomography for selecting patients with bullous lung disease for surgery. Thorax 1986;41(11):855–62.
50. Fiore D, Biondetti PR, Sartori F, et al. The role of computed tomography in the evaluation of bullous lung disease. J Comput Assist Tomogr 1982;6(1):105–8.
51. Baldwin ED, Cournand A, Richards DW Jr. Pulmonary insufficiency; a study of 122 cases of chronic pulmonary emphysema. Medicine (Baltimore) 1949;28(2):201–37.
52. Hugh-Jones P, Lambert AV. A simple standard exercise test and its use for measuring exertion dyspnoea. Br Med J 1952;1(4749):65–71.
53. Surveillance for respiratory hazards in the occupational setting [American Thoracic Society]. Am Rev Respir Dis 1982;126(5):952–6.
54. Deslauriers J. A perspective on the role of surgery in chronic obstructive lung disease. Chest Surg Clin N Am 1995;5(4):575–602.
55. Billig DM, Boushy SF, Kohen R. Surgical treatment of bullous emphysema. Arch Surg 1968;97(5):744–9.
56. Lopez-Majano V, Kieffer RF Jr, Marine DN, et al. Pulmonary resection in bullous disease. Am Rev Respir Dis 1969;99(4):554–64.
57. Berry BE, Ochsner A Jr. Massive hemoptysis associated with localized pulmonary bullae requiring emergency surgery. A case report. J Thorac Cardiovasc Surg 1972;63(1):94–8.
58. Dartevelle P, Macchiarini P, Chapelier A. Operative technique of bullectomy. Chest Surg Clin N Am 1995;5(4):735–49.
59. Cooper JD. Technique to reduce air leaks after resection of emphysematous lung. Ann Thorac Surg 1994;57(4):1038–9.

60. Miller JI Jr, Landreneau RJ, Wright CE, et al. A comparative study of buttressed versus nonbuttressed staple line in pulmonary resections. Ann Thorac Surg 2001; 71(1):319–22 [discussion: 323].
61. Stammberger U, Klepetko W, Stamatis G, et al. Buttressing the staple line in lung volume reduction surgery: a randomized three-center study. Ann Thorac Surg 2000;70(6):1820–5.
62. Murray KD, Ho CH, Hsia JY, et al. The influence of pulmonary staple line reinforcement on air leaks. Chest 2002;122(6):2146–9.
63. Weissberg D. Bullous emphysema: guidelines for management and results of operative treatment. Bronchopneumologie 1980;30(3):198–201.
64. Wakabayashi A. Thoracoscopic technique for management of giant bullous lung disease. Ann Thorac Surg 1993;56(3):708–12.
65. Yim AP, Liu HP, Hazelrigg SR, et al. Thoracoscopic operations on reoperated chests. Ann Thorac Surg 1998;65(2):328–30.
66. Macarthur AM, Fountain SW. Intracavity suction and drainage in the treatment of emphysematous bullae. Thorax 1977;32(6):668–72.
67. Goldstraw P, Petrou M. The surgical treatment of emphysema. The Brompton approach. Chest Surg Clin N Am 1995;5(4):777–96.
68. Vigneswaran WT, Townsend ER, Fountain SW. Surgery for bullous disease of the lung. Eur J Cardiothorac Surg 1992;6(8):427–30.
69. Shah SS, Goldstraw P. Surgical treatment of bullous emphysema: experience with the Brompton technique. Ann Thorac Surg 1994;58(5):1452–6.
70. Pearson MG, Ogilvie C. Surgical treatment of emphysematous bullae: late outcome. Thorax 1983;38(2):134–7.
71. Laros CD, Gelissen HJ, Bergstein PG, et al. Bullectomy for giant bullae in emphysema. J Thorac Cardiovasc Surg 1986;91(1):63–70.
72. Vejlsted H, Halkier E. Surgical improvement of patients with pulmonary insufficiency due to localized bullous emphysema or giant cysts. Thorac Cardiovasc Surg 1985;33(6):335–6.
73. Schipper PH, Meyers BF, Battafarano RJ, et al. Outcomes after resection of giant emphysematous bullae. Ann Thorac Surg 2004;78(3):976–82 [discussion: 976–82].
74. Palla A, Desideri M, Rossi G, et al. Elective surgery for giant bullous emphysema: a 5-year clinical and functional follow-up. Chest 2005;128(4):2043–50.
75. De Giacomo T, Venuta F, Rendina EA, et al. Video-assisted thoracoscopic treatment of giant bullae associated with emphysema. Eur J Cardiothorac Surg 1999; 15(6):753–6 [discussion: 756–7].
76. Rena O, Papalia E, Mineo TC, et al. Air-leak management after upper lobectomy in patients with fused fissure and chronic obstructive pulmonary disease: a pilot trial comparing sealant and standard treatment. Interact Cardiovasc Thorac Surg 2009;9(6):973–7.
77. Tambiah J, Rawlins R, Robb D, et al. Can tissue adhesives and glues significantly reduce the incidence and length of postoperative air leaks in patients having lung resections? Interact Cardiovasc Thorac Surg 2007;6(4):529–33.
78. Serra-Mitjans M, Belda-Sanchis J, Rami-Porta R. Surgical sealant for preventing air leaks after pulmonary resections in patients with lung cancer. Cochrane Database Syst Rev 2005;3:CD003051.
79. Moser C, Opitz I, Zhai W, et al. Autologous fibrin sealant reduces the incidence of prolonged air leak and duration of chest tube drainage after lung volume reduction surgery: a prospective randomized blinded study. J Thorac Cardiovasc Surg 2008;136(4):843–9.

80. Cerfolio RJ, Bass C, Katholi CR. Prospective randomized trial compares suction versus water seal for air leaks. Ann Thorac Surg 2001;71(5):1613–7.

81. Cooper JD, Trulock EP, Triantafillou AN, et al. Bilateral pneumectomy (volume reduction) for chronic obstructive pulmonary disease. J Thorac Cardiovasc Surg 1995;109(1):106–16 [discussion: 116–9].

82. McKenna RJ Jr, Benditt JO, DeCamp M, et al. Safety and efficacy of median sternotomy versus video-assisted thoracic surgery for lung volume reduction surgery. J Thorac Cardiovasc Surg 2004;127(5):1350–60.

83. Rationale and design of the National Emphysema Treatment Trial (NETT). A prospective randomized trial of lung volume reduction surgery. J Thorac Cardiovasc Surg 1999;118(3):518–28.

84. Yusen RD, Lefrak SS, Gierada DS, et al. A prospective evaluation of lung volume reduction surgery in 200 consecutive patients. Chest 2003;123(4):1026–37.

85. Ries AL, Make BJ, Lee SM, et al. The effects of pulmonary rehabilitation in the national emphysema treatment trial. Chest 2005;128(6):3799–809.

86. Naunheim KS, Wood DE, Mohsenifar Z, et al. Long-term follow-up of patients receiving lung-volume-reduction surgery versus medical therapy for severe emphysema by the National Emphysema Treatment Trial Research Group. Ann Thorac Surg 2006;82(2):431–43.

87. Pompeo E, Sergiacomi G, Nofroni I, et al. Morphologic grading of emphysema is useful in the selection of candidates for unilateral or bilateral reduction pneumoplasty. Eur J Cardiothorac Surg 2000;17(6):680–6.

88. Gierada DS, Yusen RD, Villanueva IA, et al. Patient selection for lung volume reduction surgery: An objective model based on prior clinical decisions and quantitative CT analysis. Chest 2000;117(4):991–8.

89. Hersh CP, Washko GR, Jacobson FL, et al. Interobserver variability in the determination of upper lobe-predominant emphysema. Chest 2007;131(2):424–31.

90. Patients at high risk of death after lung-volume-reduction surgery. N Engl J Med 2001;345(15):1075–83.

91. Meyers BF, Yusen RD, Guthrie TJ, et al. Results of lung volume reduction surgery in patients meeting a national emphysema treatment trial high-risk criterion. J Thorac Cardiovasc Surg 2004;127(3):829–35.

92. Ciccone AM, Meyers BF, Guthrie TJ, et al. Long-term outcome of bilateral lung volume reduction in 250 consecutive patients with emphysema. J Thorac Cardiovasc Surg 2003;125(3):513–25.

93. Patel N, DeCamp M, Criner GJ. Lung transplantation and lung volume reduction surgery versus transplantation in chronic obstructive pulmonary disease. Proc Am Thorac Soc 2008;5(4):447–53.

94. Christie JD, Edwards LB, Aurora P, et al. Registry of the International Society for Heart and Lung Transplantation: twenty-fifth official adult lung and heart/lung transplantation report–2008. J Heart Lung Transplant 2008;27(9):957–69.

The Diaphragm

Mary S. Maish, MD, MPH

KEYWORDS

• Diaphragm • Solitary fibrous tumor • Phrenic nerve
• Diaphragmatic hernia • Eventration

Although the diaphragm is not so grandiose, without it life as it is currently known would not be possible. This then begs the question, when did the diaphragm first develop and for what purpose? As it turns out this is a matter of semantics. As far back as 300 million years ago, vertebrate species had a primitive diaphragm that served only to separate an upper feeding compartment from a lower digestive tract.[1] In dinosaurs and other reptile and amphibious species, the lungs were always caudal to the diaphragm. Not until warm-blooded mammals evolved did the lungs herniate through the diaphragm into the thoracic cavity and became a critical component of respiratory function.[2] This transition is thought to have occurred about 100 million years ago in rodent type mammals. The diaphragm is now a critical organ for proper respiration and is present in some form in more than 5000 mammalian species. The diaphragm may be subtle in its presence but is indispensible in its function.

EMBRYOLOGY

The development of the diaphragm begins in the seventh week of gestation and is complete by the tenth week. It is derived from four embryologic precursors: the septum transversum, the right and left pleuroperitoneal membranes, and the dorsal mesentery of the esophagus (**Fig. 1**). The septum transversum is an anterior structure that becomes the central tendon and fuses with three dorsal structures to form the primitive diaphragm. The dorsal mesentery, containing the primitive aorta, inferior vena cava, and esophagus, becomes the posteromedial portion of the diaphragm. Myoblasts migrate into this structure, forming the crura bilaterally. The right and left pleuroperitoneal membranes grow medially and anteriorly to fuse with the central tendon. The final phase of diaphragmatic development is the formation of the neuro-muscular component. The muscle fibers migrate from the third, fourth, and fifth cervical myotomes of the body wall. The phrenic nerves arising from the third, fourth, and fifth cervical nerves migrate distally, completing the final phase of diaphragmatic development.[3]

Disclosures: The author has nothing to disclose.
Department of Surgery, UCLA David Geffen School of Medicine, 10833 Le Conte Avenue, Room 64-124 CHS, Box 957313, Los Angeles, CA 90095-7313, USA
E-mail address: mmaish@mednet.ucla.edu

Surg Clin N Am 90 (2010) 955–968
doi:10.1016/j.suc.2010.07.005
0039-6109/10/$ – see front matter © 2010 Elsevier Inc. All rights reserved.

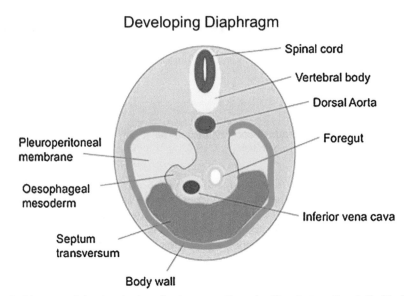

Developing Diaphragm

Spinal cord

Vertebral body

Dorsal Aorta

Foregut

Pleuroperitoneal membrane

Oesophageal mesoderm

Septum transversum

Inferior vena cava

Body wall

Fig. 1. Diagram of the developing diaphragm at 7 weeks. (Respiratory Dev © Dr Mark Hill 2008 Slide 30; Available at: http://embryology.med.unsw.edu.au. Accessed June 1, 2010; with permission.)

The importance of understanding embryologic development for a surgeon lies in gaining an understanding of the common variants and uncommon congenital defects that are encountered in surgical practice. Fortunately, the diaphragm is a very consistent organ and has no normal variations. However, several common abnormalities result from faulty embryologic development, including congenital diaphragmatic hernias and eventration, which will be addressed later.

ANATOMY

The Greek derivation of the words *dia* (in between) and *phragma* (fence) aptly describes this organ. The diaphragm is a musculofibrous dome-shaped membrane that separates the thoracic from the abdominal cavity. It has a muscular portion peripherally, and a fibrous portion centrally (**Fig. 2**). It has three major muscle groups: sternal, costal, and lumbar and a large fibrinous central tendon composed of three leaflets: right, left, and middle. Major structures pass through three openings: the caval opening (T8), the esophageal hiatus (T10), and the aortic hiatus (T12). In addition to the aorta, the aortic hiatus also allows passage for the thoracic duct and the azygos vein. The muscle origins are from the sternum anteriorly, the lower six ribs laterally, and the arcuate ligaments posteriorly. The crura are posterior muscle bundles that arise from the lumbar vertebrae: the right from L1–3 and the left from L1–2.[4]

BLOOD SUPPLY

The major arterial blood supply to the diaphragm comes from the left and right phrenic arteries (see **Fig. 2**). These paired arteries arise directly from the abdominal aorta near the aortic hiatus. They bifurcate posteriorly and give off a large anterior branch, which courses along the anterior and superior portions of the muscle, merging with the

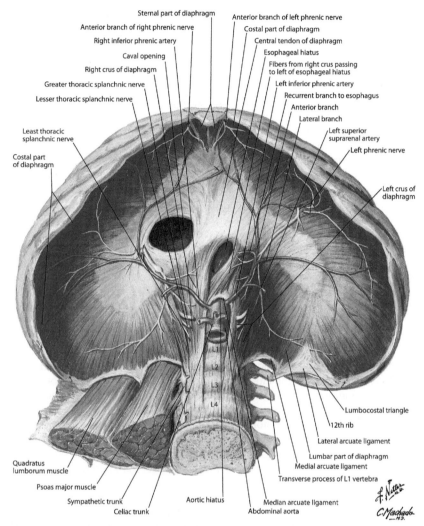

Sternal part of diaphragm
Anterior branch of right phrenic nerve
Right inferior phrenic artery
Caval opening
Right crus of diaphragm
Greater thoracic splanchnic nerve
Lesser thoracic splanchnic nerve
Least thoracic splanchnic nerve
Costal part of diaphragm

Anterior branch of left phrenic nerve
Costal part of diaphragm
Central tendon of diaphragm
Esophageal hiatus
Fibers from right crus passing to left of esophageal hiatus
Left inferior phrenic artery
Recurrent branch to esophagus
Anterior branch
Lateral branch
Left superior suprarenal artery
Left phrenic nerve
Left crus of diaphragm

L1
L2
L3
L4

Lumbocostal triangle
12th rib
Lateral arcuate ligament
Lumbar part of diaphragm
Medial arcuate ligament
Transverse process of L1 vertebra

Quadratus lumborum muscle
Psoas major muscle
Sympathetic trunk
Celiac trunk
Aortic hiatus
Median arcuate ligament
Abdominal aorta

Fig. 2. Anatomy of the diaphragm. (*From* www.netterimages.com. Accessed June 1, 2010. © Elsevier Inc. All rights reserved; with permission.)

pericardiophrenic artery. Additional arterial blood is supplied to the diaphragm from branches off of the right and left internal mammary arteries.

The venous drainage is consistent and is via the right and left inferior phrenic veins. These veins run alongside the arteries and drain medially into the inferior vena cava. All of the vascular structures are best seen from the abdomen.

INNERVATION

The diaphragm is innervated exclusively from the right and left phrenic nerves that originate from C3–4–5. These paired nerves provide both sensory and motor function to the diaphragm. The phrenic nerve traverses the thoracic cavity posteriorly and moves anterior over the pericardium. The right phrenic nerve pierces the diaphragm just lateral to the caval hiatus, and the left pierces just lateral to the left heart border.

Each nerve divides into four trunks: an anterolateral, posterolateral, sternal, and crural trunk (see **Fig. 2**). After giving off the sternal branch, the nerves penetrate the diaphragm and course along inferiorly and are, again, best seen from the abdomen.

FUNCTION

The principle function of the diaphragm is breathing: inhalation and exhalation. During inhalation the diaphragm contracts. With the aid of the external intercostal muscles, the thoracic cavity expands, reducing intrathoracic pressure and allowing air to rush into the lungs. When the diaphragm relaxes, the elastic recoil allows air to be drawn out passively from the lungs. For optimum respiratory function, both hemidiaphragms must be intact. Injury to one phrenic nerve results in an elevated hemidiaphragm and impaired respiratory mechanics. Injury to both phrenic nerves results in near-apnea, resulting in heavy recruitment of accessory muscles of respiration that can compensate only in the short term.

Although the diaphragm is generally under involuntary neural control from the central nervous system, it can be augmented by voluntary input.[5] The diaphragm also has nonrespiratory functions, including separation of the abdominal and thoracic cavity, helping to expel vomit, feces, and urine from the body through increasing intra-abdominal pressure and preventing acid reflux through exerting pressure on the lower esophageal sphincter.

SURGICAL CONSIDERATIONS

Preservation of at least one phrenic nerve is critical during any surgical procedure. The nerve courses posteriorly in the lateral compartment of the neck and can be inadvertently injured during posterior neck dissections. As it courses through the thoracic cavity, it transitions from a posterior to anterior position and can be seen on the anterior surface of the pericardium before it pierces the diaphragm. Care must be taken to identify the course of the nerve before opening the pericardium. The nerve is often involved in tumors of the chest wall and mediastinum, and may need to be sacrificed. More commonly, the nerve is drawn up toward the tumor from peritumoral inflammation and may be salvageable with careful, often tedious dissection of the nerve away from the bulky tumor.

When opening of the diaphragm is necessary, for either access or excision of the muscle, an understanding of how the nerve traverses across the diaphragm is helpful. **Fig. 3** shows the course of the nerve and where incisions should be placed to preserve nerve function. Circumferential incisions should be placed parallel to the edge of the muscle to avoid nerve injury. Radial incisions traverse from the central tendon outward toward the chest wall and should be placed so that only the distal branches of the nerve are transected. Combinations of these two types of incisions should be used to achieve adequate exposure.

The diaphragm itself can be accessed through an abdominal or thoracic approach. An upper midline, subcostal, or chevron incision is best used to access the diaphragm from the abdomen. From this vantage point, both leaves of the diaphragms can be visualized. Because of its juxtaposition to the liver, the posterior right hemidiaphragm is difficult to access from this side. The entire left hemidiaphragm is easily viewed through an abdominal exposure. To obtain exposure of the diaphragm through a thoracic incision, the thoracotomy is performed at or below the sixth intercostal space. An anterolateral incision is made when access to the esophageal hiatus is needed, such as for the repair of a paraesophageal hernia. A posterolateral incision

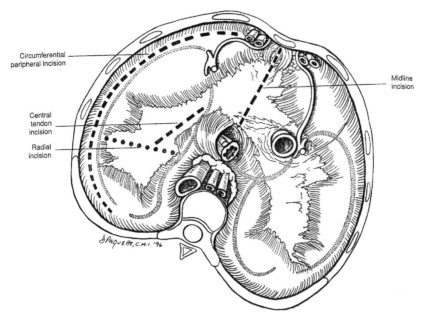

Fig. 3. Diaphragmatic incisions. (*From* Daly BD, Feins NR. The diaphragm. In: Kaiser LR, Kron IL, Spray TL, editors. Mastery of cardiothoracic surgery. Philadelphia (PA): Lippincott-Raven, Lippincott, Williams and Wilkins; 1998. p. 200; with permission.)

is made when access to the posterior diaphragm is needed, such as for traumatic and congenital diaphragmatic hernias.

Although the diaphragm can be completely removed, reconstruction is necessary to preserve intrathoracic mechanics and respiratory function. When the hemidiaphragm, either a portion or in its entirety, needs to be resected, reconstruction can be performed without a prosthetic patch.[6] Nonabsorbable mesh with a smooth surface (to abut up against the lung) is best. Various materials accomplish these goals, including polypropylene mesh, woven polytetrafluoroethylene (PTFE) or GORE-TEX (W. L. Gore and Associates, Elkton, MA, USA) mesh, bovine pericardium, Surgisis (Cook Medical, Bloomington, IN, USA), and polyester PTFE patch. Heavy nonabsorbable sutures placed in a mattress fashion are used for securing the patch to the diaphragm.

Repair is performed with consideration to preservation of the phrenic nerve, whereas reconstruction requires an understanding of the origin and insertion of the diaphragm muscles as described earlier. Peripherally the mesh is sewn to the chest wall: the sternum anteriorly, the ribs laterally, and the prevertebral fascia posteriorly. In the absence of the central tendon, the mesh is approximated to the midline organs and soft tissues, medially, with absorbable sutures placed in an interrupted fashion.

IMAGING AND TESTING

Many pathologic conditions affect the diaphragm, both anatomically and functionally. Precise localization and characterization of tumors and diaphragmatic injury may be necessary, and identifying functional abnormalities before and after surgery is often helpful. Chest radiography is a useful screening tool for diaphragmatic abnormalities.[7] Hernia defects and functional defects can be seen easily. Cross-sectional imaging with ultrasound,[8] high-resolution CT, and MRI can illustrate intrinsic pathology and assist in the evaluation of peridiaphragmatic masses.[9] The latter two modalities, especially, clearly delineate the complex anatomic relationships that the diaphragm shares with major intrathoracic and intra-abdominal organs.[7] MRI has the added advantage of showing relationships of the diaphragm to neurovascular structures.

Fluoroscopy is used primarily to evaluate diaphragmatic motion. The sniff test is a fluoroscopic examination used to evaluate the function of the diaphragm during a cycle of respiration.[10] While performing dynamic imaging of the diaphragm, the radiologist will ask the patient to sniff, or quickly breathe in through the nose. This maneuver exaggerates the difference in a paralyzed hemidiaphragm, which will move paradoxically in a cephalad direction. Cine-MRI is also used to evaluate diaphragmatic motion access degrees of diaphragmatic paresis.

Electromyography of the diaphragm elicited by phrenic nerve stimulation provides useful information on diaphragm function and for the diagnosis of neuromuscular disorders. Electrical stimulation of the phrenic nerve via an esophageal electrode facilitates the measurement of phrenic nerve conduction time. Newer techniques using cervical magnetic stimulation are also being used to accurately access diaphragmatic function.[11]

CONGENITAL DEFECTS OF THE DIAPHRAGM
Hernia of Morgagni

Giovanni Battista Morgagni was an Italian anatomist, celebrated as the father of modern anatomic pathology. In 1769 he described an anterior retrosternal diaphragmatic defect that occurs between the xiphoid process of the sternum and costochondral attachments of the diaphragm (**Fig. 4**). It results from failure of muscle tissue to spread over the area during embryologic development and constitutes less than 2% of reported diaphragmatic defects.[12] Because the space is covered by pericardium on the left, abdominal contents more commonly herniate through the defect on the right. The hernia usually has a sac unless it has ruptured in prenatal life, which can often be determined by a prenatal ultrasound.[13] Although it is congenital, it is rarely noticed in children and most often is found in adults presenting with fullness and cramping.[14] It is seen more commonly in women and obese individuals. Frequently, it is an incidental finding found on a screening chest radiograph for some other condition. CT scanning is used to image the defect and evaluate the extent of abdominal visceral herniation, whereas an upper gastrointestinal series is used to identify the contents of the hernia sac.[12]

Surgical correction of a hernia of Morgagni is undertaken at initial diagnosis and even in the absence of symptoms.[15] Neglect can lead to bowel obstruction, ischemia, and necrosis in some cases. Observation is reserved for debilitated patients. Patients are prepared for surgery with a liquid diet for 24-hours in advance. A complete bowel preparation is not necessary. A nasogastric tube is placed to help with bowel decompression. The repair is performed using an abdominal approach: either an upper midline or subcostal incision. Laparoscopic approaches have also been undertaken with success.[16]

Transthoracic repair is appropriate when the contents of the hernia are fixed in position at or above the level of the carina. Reduction of these structures can be difficult using the abdominal approach because of dense adhesions, and so a transthoracic approach is preferred under these circumstances. The hernia sac is identified, its contents are reduced, and the sac is resected. The defect in the diaphragm is evaluated for size and location. Small defects that are surrounded entirely by a rim of muscle may be repaired primarily with heavy nonabsorbable interrupted mattress sutures (**Fig. 5**A). A defect with an incomplete muscular rim is repaired by attaching the free edge of the muscle to the costal margin (see **Fig. 5**B). Defects that are too

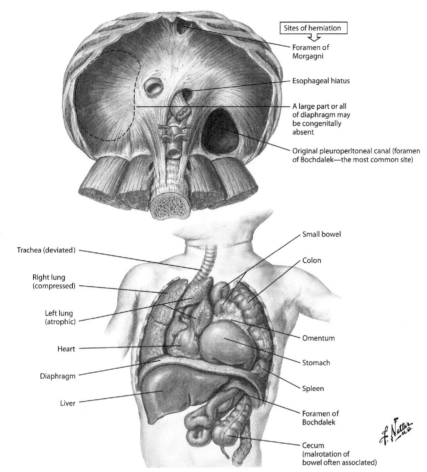

Sites of herniation

Foramen of Morgagni

Esophageal hiatus

A large part or all of diaphragm may be congenitally absent

Original pleuroperitoneal canal (foramen of Bochdalek—the most common site)

Trachea (deviated)

Right lung (compressed)

Left lung (atrophic)

Heart

Diaphragm

Liver

Small bowel

Colon

Omentum

Stomach

Spleen

Foramen of Bochdalek

Cecum (malrotation of bowel often associated)

Fig. 4. Hernia of Morgagni. Congenital Diaphragmatic Hernias. (*From* www.netterimages. com. Accessed June 1, 2010. © Elsevier Inc. All rights reserved.)

large to close primarily without resulting tension should be closed with a nonabsorbable mesh interposed between the muscular rim and the chest wall. A chest tube is placed and the wound is closed.

Hernia of Bochdalek

Vincenz Alexander Bochdalek, a Czech anatomist living in the 19th century, first described this congenital diaphragmatic hernia as a defect occurring during early embryologic development. During this phase, the gut is formed and, because of abnormal development, the viscera are trapped in the chest, preventing adequate formation of the lungs and resulting in pulmonary hypoplasia. Up to 85% of neonates born with this condition will be in critical condition at delivery,[17] and up to 60% will not survive past the neonatal period.[18] Bochdalek's hernia constitutes 90% of all diaphragmatic hernias and occurs in approximately 1 of every 2200 to 12,500 births every year.[19] In contrast to hernias of Morgagni, these defects are commonly associated with other congenital abnormalities, especially those that are cardiac in nature. They

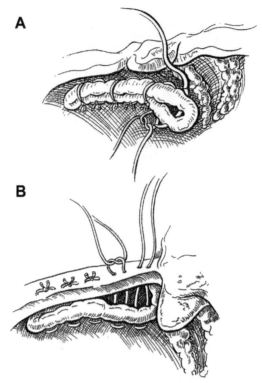

Fig. 5. Repair of a Hernia of Morgagni. (*A*) Anterior rim of tissue is present. (*B*) Anterior rim of tissue is absent. (*From* Daly BD, Feins NR. The diaphragm. In: Kaiser LR, Kron IL, Spray TL, editors. Mastery of cardiothoracic surgery. Philadelphia (PA): Lippincott-Raven, Lippincott, Williams and Wilkins; 1998. p. 203; with permission.)

occur more commonly in men than women, by a ratio of 3:2, and are left-sided 85% of the time (see **Fig. 4**).

The diagnosis is usually made with a prenatal ultrasound.[20] After delivery, the infant is supported by mechanical ventilation until repair is undertaken. Mechanical ventilation alone can often restore adequate gas exchange so that surgery can be delayed. Extracorporeal membrane oxygenation (ECMO) is used in infants for whom mechanical ventilation is unsatisfactory. ECMO is often sustained until the infant is decannulated after surgical repair, but this is institution biased.[21,22] Often other defects must be emergently addressed in an operative setting, and the hernia is repaired simultaneously. In other instances, emergent repair is not necessary, and aggressive neonatal resuscitation has proven to be beneficial in the survival of these infants. Despite early diagnosis and advanced intensive care management, the operative mortality approaches 50%.[23]

At repair, a subcostal transverse incision is made leaving 2 to 3 cm between the incision and the costal margin. Good retraction affords a view of the defect in its entirety. The hernia sac (present up to 20% of the time) is identified, its contents carefully reduced, and its walls resected. The posterior lip of the defect is identified above the adrenal gland and freed for closure. In some cases a primary closure can be undertaken. When not enough tissue is available, the defect is closed with a patch that is secured to the ribs with nonabsorbable interrupted sutures over Teflon pledgets.[22]

After the diaphragmatic defect is closed, the visceral organs are returned to the abdomen. To prevent abdominal compartment syndrome, a ventral hernia or silo may need to be created to accommodate all of the organs. A chest tube is attached to an underwater seal to prevent further lung damage. Cardiomyopathy and renal failure are common in the postoperative period, and chronic bronchopulmonary dysplasia, mental retardation, and neurologic deficits are common in the long term.

ACQUIRED DEFECTS OF THE DIAPHRAGM
Acute Diaphragmatic Hernias

The most common cause of an acquired diaphragmatic hernia is blunt or penetrating trauma. Motor vehicle accidents are the leading cause of blunt diaphragmatic injury, whereas penetrating injuries result from gunshot or stab wounds. Among patients admitted to the hospital for trauma, 3% to 5% have a diaphragmatic hernia.[24] They occur more commonly in men than women, at a ratio of 4:1, with most presenting in the third decade of life. Upwards of 75% of patients have tears from penetrating injuries, whereas fewer than 2% of patients have rupture from blunt injuries. Approximately 69% of hernias are left-sided, 24% are right-sided, and 15% are bilateral. Nonetheless, blunt injuries are far more common and account for 75% of acquired defects.[25] Other rare causes of traumatic rupture include labor in women who have had prior diaphragmatic hernia repair[26] and barotrauma during scuba diving in patients with a history of nissen fundoplication.[27]

Acquired diaphragmatic hernias affect physiology in many ways. Circulatory and respiratory depression occur as a result of decreased diaphragmatic function, compression of the lungs from intra-abdominal contents, shifting of the mediastinum, and cardiac compromise. Smaller diaphragmatic hernias are often not discovered until months or years later, when patients present with strangulation of intra-abdominal organs, dyspnea, or nonspecific gastrointestinal complaints.

In the acute setting, patients present with respiratory distress, decreased breath sounds on the affected side, auscultation of bowel sounds in the chest, palpation of abdominal contents during insertion of a chest tube, paradoxic motion of the abdomen with breathing, or abdominal pain. Patients often present asymptomatically or have distraction injuries. Increased clinical acumen by the treating physician is necessary to detect this injury.

Traumatic rupture of the diaphragm requires surgical intervention whether the patient presents immediately or sometime after the trauma. Repair of the acute diaphragmatic rupture from trauma is directed by other injuries that may be present. In the absence of intrathoracic injuries, the high incidence of concomitant intra-abdominal injuries dictates the need for emergency abdominal exploration in the acute trauma setting after initial resuscitation is accomplished. Before induction of anesthesia, a nasogastric tube should be inserted to help bowel decompression and reduce the chance of aspiration on induction. A midline incision is made so that a complete abdominal exploration is possible. Critical injuries are controlled and the diaphragmatic defect is assessed for size and viability. Areas of nonviable tissue are resected. Small defects are closed primarily with interrupted horizontal mattress sutures. Larger defects are patched with mesh. A running suture may be used to approximate the mesh to the central tendon. When nerve injury has occurred and functional impairment is imminent, the mesh repair should be taut to prevent paradoxic movement.

Chronic Diaphragmatic Hernias

Chronic diaphragmatic hernias are acquired defects that remain asymptomatic for months to years after initial injury. Patients who present in the latent phase or long after trauma require repair because the hernia contents may become strangulated, leading to ischemia or necrosis of the gut, stomach, liver, spleen, or other organs. The surgical approach has traditionally been through a thoracotomy incision in the 7th or 8th intercostal space. With the advent of video-assisted surgery, however, laparoscopic and thoracoscopic repair is acceptable. Thoracoscopic repair should be reserved for small defects, because the contents of a large hernia will obscure an adequate view. If preoperative imaging shows hernia contents above the level of the inferior pulmonary vein, an intrathoracic approach is preferred and safest. Unlike acute hernias, chronic hernias form dense adhesions to surrounding structures that are difficult and unsafe to divide using an abdominal approach. The principles involved in the surgery are reduction of hernia contents back into the abdomen, excision of the entire hernia sac, and repair of the diaphragmatic defect. Small defects may be repaired primarily, whereas large defects should be closed with a mesh patch to avoid tension on the repair and postoperative disruption.

If a thoracoscopic approach is planned, the patient is placed into the lateral decubitus position with single lung ventilation secured. A camera port is placed into the midaxillary line at the 4th intercostal space. Two additional ports are placed strategically to triangulate onto the dome of the diaphragm: one posterior to and one anterior to the midaxillary line. Once the hernia sac is reduced, a moist laparotomy sponge can be placed through the diaphragm to keep the abdominal contents reduced while closure is underway. It is then removed before securing the final sutures.

The laparoscopic approach requires a camera port just above the umbilicus in the midline. For left-sided defects, a Nathanson liver retractor is placed just below the xiphoid process and two working ports are placed into the right and left subcostal positions. For right-sided defects, a paddle liver retractor is placed in the right lower quadrant and working ports are placed into the left subcostal and left paraumbilical positions. Additional ports may need to be placed to help reduce the hernia sac and enable adequate visualization during the repair.

EVENTRATION OF THE DIAPHRAGM

The broader definition of *eventration* is the abnormal elevation of the hemidiaphragm. It can be classified into congenital and acquired forms. The acquired form is usually caused by phrenic nerve injury and is reviewed in the next section. In the strictest sense, however, eventration refers to the congenital abnormality that occurs from failure of the fetal diaphragm to muscularize.[28] A narrow rim of muscle is present peripherally that contracts with electrical stimulation, resulting in a thin, pliable central portion of the hemidiaphragm. It is frequently associated with other congenital abnormalities of the spine and chest, hypoplastic lungs, extrapulmonary sequestration, and transposition of the viscera. Children born with this defect are often in cardiopulmonary distress and on mechanical ventilation or ECMO. In these infants, immediate repair is undertaken. Delayed repair is safe for infants who are not in extremis.

Whether congenital or acquired, repair of diaphragmatic eventration is best performed through a thoracotomy incision in the 7th or 8th intercostal space. The goal of the operation is to tighten the diaphragm and restore it close to its intended anatomic location.[29] The diaphragm is incised near its costal attachments and stretched out. It is reattached with interrupted nonabsorbable sutures placed in a horizontal mattress fashion. Thoracoscopic repair is gaining favor. A 10-mm camera port is placed in the 5th intercostal space posteriorly and a 5-mm port is placed in the 5th intercostal space anteriorly. A mini-thoracotomy incision is made over the 9th or 10th intercostal space. First, a running suture is used to invaginate the eventration.

A second running suture is then used over the top of the first to adjust to the desired tension. Other thoracoscopic and laparoscopic techniques have been described to avoid the mini-thoracotomy[6]; however, the principles of repair remain the same.

DIAPHRAGMATIC PARALYSIS

Diaphragmatic paralysis can result from direct injury to the diaphragm or injury to the phrenic nerve. In infants, direct injury is most common during cardiac surgery and can result in life-threatening respiratory insufficiency. This condition has been attributed to three factors: weak intercostal muscles preventing a significant increase in intrathoracic dimensions, a mobile mediastinum shifting away from the paralyzed side during inspiration limiting lung expansion, and a tendency toward recumbency wherein the abdominal viscera exert undue force in an upward direction.[22] Early assessment of diaphragm function is performed at the bedside for intubated patients. In children younger than 18 months, the current recommendation is to perform diaphragmatic plication within 2 weeks of diagnosis. In children older than 18 months, plication is generally not necessary.

Diaphragmatic plication in a child is performed using the technique originally described by Schwartz and Filler[30] in 1978. The diaphragm is plicated centrally with interrupted 3-0 horizontal mattress sutures buttressed with Teflon pledgets, spaced 0.5 cm apart. The sutures are deliberately placed into the muscle between the branches of the phrenic nerve. Commonly, diaphragmatic function returns after some time.

In adults, diaphragmatic injury almost always occurs on the left side and is attributed to hypothermia during cardiopulmonary arrest. The overall incidence is approximately 2% and is more commonly associated with open procedures and reoperations. Most often the paralysis is temporary. Paralysis may also result from direct invasion of the phrenic nerve by tumors of the lung and mediastinum and trauma associated with sudden deceleration. In these instances, paralysis is often permanent. Paralysis has also been associated with neuromuscular disorders, difficult births, cervical osteoarthritis, a substernal thyroid, an aortic aneurysm, von Recklinghausen disease, Lyme disease, and viral, bacterial, syphilitic, and tuberculous infections. Noncardiac thoracic or cervical operations also may cause paralysis from direct injury to the nerve, traction on the nerve, pressure from a retractor, or use of cautery near the nerve.

Unilateral diaphragmatic paralysis is not associated with a significant respiratory dysfunction in most patients, but can lead to dyspnea and affect ventilatory function. An initial reduction in vital capacity and total lung capacity of 20% to 30% usually returns to normal after 6 months. It has been documented that most patients reporting an initial symptom of cough or chest pain experienced improvement of these symptoms on follow-up, whereas in two thirds of patients whose primary complaint was dyspnea on exertion, these symptoms remained unchanged or deteriorated.[31] The prognosis is usually good in unilateral paralysis in the absence of neurologic or pulmonary processes. Patients with bilateral paralysis, although rare, present with marked reduction in vital capacity and flow rates and may show excessive accessory muscle movement. The prognosis for patients with bilateral paralysis is usually poor and often leads to long-term mechanical ventilation through a permanent tracheostomy.

In adults, diaphragmatic plication should be considered in symptomatic patients whose phrenic nerve has irreversible injury, generally after 1 year. Plication alters the shape of the diaphragm and allows vital capacity and lung capacity to increase. These increases can continue for up to a year, along with increases in residual volume, diffusing capacity, and partial arterial oxygen.[32] A thoracotomy through the 7th or 8th intercostal space is recommended. The lateral and posterior portions of the diaphragm are gathered in pleats and sutured with interrupted, pledgeted, horizontal mattress sutures.[33] Thoracoscopic repair has also been described, although long-term results are not well studied.[34]

DIAPHRAGMATIC PACING

There are few indications for diaphragmatic pacing. Patients with central alveolar hypoventilation (Ondine's curse) and those with high cervical cord injuries (quadriplegics) may benefit.[35] Although it has been used in patients with chronic obstructive pulmonary disease, intractable hiccups, and phrenic nerve injury, it has no proven benefits in these conditions.

Central alveolar hypoventilation is caused by a lack of response to hypercarbia and hypoxia during sleep by the receptors in the medulla. Pacing the diaphragm allows these patients to sleep while continuing to breathe even in the absence of central nervous system stimulation. High cervical spine injuries (above C3) are most amenable to phrenic nerve pacing because the nerve is still intact.[36] In these patients, diaphragmatic pacing decreases the need for mechanical ventilation.

The electrode is placed under general anesthesia through a limited anterior thoracotomy. The phrenic nerve is indentified at the mid-sternal level. An electrode is placed flat against the mediastinum and underneath the phrenic nerve. The other end is connected to a receiver unit that is placed in a subcutaneous pocket. If both sides need to be addressed, the surgeries are staged several weeks apart.

DIAPHRAGMATIC TUMORS

Primary diaphragmatic tumors are rare and most are benign. Benign lesions include lipomas, fibromas, schwannomas, neurofibromas, leiomyomas, and bronchial, mesothelial, echinococcal, or teratogenous cysts. Malignant diaphragmatic tumors include solitary fibrous tumors and fibrosarcomas, which are the most common. Much more common than primary diaphragmatic tumors is direct invasion of the diaphragm by a tumor arising in an adjacent structure, such as a lower lobe bronchogenic carcinoma, mesothelioma, or tumors of the stomach, pleura, chest wall, mediastinum, liver, or esophagus.[37]

Benign lesions are generally asymptomatic, but when symptoms occur they are usually nonspecific. Often they are discovered incidentally on chest imaging. CT scans are used for imaging tumors of the diaphragm and may even reveal the origin of the mass. However, the relationship of the mass to the diaphragm is best revealed on coronal MRI images or transabdominal ultrasound. Fibrosarcomas appear as focal extrapulmonary masses that obscure all or part of the hemidiaphragm and are often indistinguishable from masses arising from within the diaphragmatic pleura. In this circumstance, MRIs are also used to clarify CT scan findings.

All tumors of the diaphragm, benign and malignant, should be resected at discovery.[37] Benign tumors just need a clear margin, whereas malignant tumors should be resected with a wide margin of normal tissue without regard to the extent of the defect. An entire leaf of the diaphragm can be removed without undue physiologic impairment. Additionally, prosthetic material can be used to repair any defects and various muscle flaps may be used to cover the defects and provide soft tissue coverage.[6] Neoadjuvant chemotherapy along with postoperative radiation therapy may be used for large tumors with positive surgical margins.

SUMMARY

This article discusses the diaphragm from a surgical perspective. Although it is a relatively simple organ compared with other structures, the diaphragm serves its host well by providing the mechanics necessary for vital respiratory function. It is replaceable in part, but as a whole it is as important as the heart and lungs, and without it the body would lack the ability to draw the wind into our sails and set our ships on course for greater adventures.

REFERENCES

1. Keith A. The nature of the mammalian diaphragm and pleural cavities. J Anat Physiol 1905;39:243–84.
2. Gibbons A. Lung fossils suggest dinos breathed in cold blood. Science 1997; 278:1229–30.
3. Schumpelick V, Steinau G, Schlüper I, et al. Surgical embryology and anatomy of the diaphragm with surgical applications [review]. Surg Clin North Am 2000; 80(1):213–39, xi.
4. Anraku M, Shargall Y. Surgical conditions of the diaphragm: anatomy and physiology [review]. Thorac Surg Clin 2009;19(4):419–29, v.
5. Kolar P, Neuwirth J, Sanda J. Analysis of diaphragm movement during tidal breathing and during its activation while breath holding using MRI synchronized with spirometry. Physiol Res 2009;58:383–92.
6. Palanivelu C, Rangarajan M, Rajapandian S, et al. Laparoscopic repair of adult diaphragmatic hernias and eventration with primary sutured closure and prosthetic reinforcement: a retrospective study. Surg Endosc 2009;23(5):978–85.
7. Mirvis SE, Shanmuganathan K. Imaging hemidiaphragmatic injury. Eur Radiol 2007;17(6):1411–21.
8. Kim SH, Na S, Choi JS, et al. An evaluation of diaphragmatic movement by M-mode sonography as a predictor of pulmonary dysfunction after upper abdominal surgery. Anesth Analg 2010;110(5):1349–54.
9. Tarver RD, Conces DJ Jr, Cory DA, et al. Imaging the diaphragm and its disorders. J Thorac Imaging 1989;4(1):1–18.
10. Roberts HC. Imaging the diaphragm. Thorac Surg Clin 2009;19(4):431–50.
11. Luo YM, Polkey MI. Diaphragm EMG measured by cervical magnetic and electrical phrenic nerve stimulation. J Appl Physiol 1998;85(6):2089–99.
12. Nasr A, Fecteau A. Foramen of Morgagni hernia: presentation and treatment [review]. Thorac Surg Clin 2009;19(4):463–8.
13. Comstock C, Bronsteen RA, Whitten A, et al. Paradoxical motion: a useful tool in the prenatal diagnosis of congenital diaphragmatic hernias and eventrations. J Ultrasound Med 2009;28(10):1365–7.
14. Schumacher L, Gilbert S. Congenital diaphragmatic hernia in the adult [review]. Thorac Surg Clin 2009;19(4):469–72.
15. Pober BR, Russell MK, Ackerman KG. Congenital diaphragmatic hernia overview [internet]. In: Pagon RA, Bird TC, Dolan CR, et al, editors. GeneReviews. Seattle (WA): University of Washington, Seattle; 1993–2006. p. 469–72.
16. Danielson PD, Chandler NM. Single-port laparoscopic repair of a Morgagni diaphragmatic hernia in a pediatric patient: advancement in single-port technology allows effective intracorporeal suturing. J Pediatr Surg 2010;45(3):E21–4.
17. Centers for Disease Control and Prevention. Hospital stays, hospital charges, and in-hospital deaths among infants with selected birth defects—United States, 2003. MMWR Morb Mortal Wkly 2007;56(2):25–9.

18. Hekmatnia A, McHugh K. Congenital diaphragmatic hernia. Available at: http://emedicine.medscape.com/article/407519-overview. Accessed February 8, 2007.
19. Keijzer R, Puri P. Congenital diaphragmatic hernia. Semin Pediatr Surg 2010; 19(3):180–5.
20. Yang JI. Left diaphragmatic eventration diagnosed as congenital diaphragmatic hernia by prenatal sonography. J Clin Ultrasound 2003;31(4):214–7.
21. Chao PH, Huang CB, Liu CA, et al. Congenital diaphragmatic hernia in the neonatal period: review of 21 years' experience. Pediatr Neonatol 2010;51(2): 97–102.
22. Lau C, Myers B. The diaphragm. In: General thoracic surgery. p. 232.
23. Hartnett KS. Congenital diaphragmatic hernia: advanced physiology and care concepts [review]. Adv Neonatal Care 2008;8(2):107–15.
24. Turhan K, Makay O, Cakan A, et al. Traumatic diaphragmatic rupture: look to see. Eur J Cardiothorac Surg 2008;33(6):1082–5.
25. Cameron JL. Diaphragmatic injury. In: Current surgical therapy. 9th edition. Philadelphia: Mosby-Elsevier; 2008. p. 975–87.
26. Hamoudi D, Bouderka MA, Benissa N, et al. Diaphragmatic rupture during labor. Int J Obstet Anesth 2004;13(4):284–6.
27. Hayden JD, Davies JB, Martin IG. Diaphragmatic rupture resulting from gastrointestinal barotrauma in a scuba diver. Br J Sports Med 1998;32(1):75–6.
28. Groth SS, Andrade RS. Diaphragmatic eventration. Thorac Surg Clin 2009;19(4): 511–9 [review].
29. Groth SS, Andrade RS. Diaphragm plication for eventration or paralysis: a review of the literature. Ann Thorac Surg 2010;89(6):S2146–50.
30. Schwartz MZ, Filler RM. Plication of the diaphragm for symptomatic phrenic nerve paralysis. J Pediatr Surg 1978;13:259–63.
31. Higgs SM, Hussain A, Jackson M, et al. Long term results of diaphragmatic plication for unilateral diaphragm paralysis. Eur J Cardiothorac Surg 2002;21(2): 294–7.
32. Freeman RK, Wozniak TC. Functional and physiologic result of video-assisted thoracoscopic diaphragm plication in adult patients with unilateral diaphragm paralysis. Ann Thorac Surg 2006;81:1853–7.
33. Mouroux J, Padovani B, Poirier NC, et al. Technique for the repair of diaphragmatic eventration. Ann Thorac Surg 1996;62(3):905–7.
34. Groth SS, Rueth NM, Kast T, et al. Laparoscopic diaphragmatic plication for diaphragmatic paralysis and eventration: an objective evaluation of short-term and midterm results. J Thorac Cardiovasc Surg 2010;139(6):1452–6.
35. DiMarco AF. Phrenic nerve stimulation in patients with spinal cord injury [review]. Respir Physiol Neurobiol 2009;169(2):200–9.
36. Sitthinamsuwan B, Nunta-aree S. Phrenic nerve stimulation for diaphragmatic pacing in a patient with high cervical spinal cord injury. J Med Assoc Thai 2009;92(12):1691–5.
37. Kim MP, Hofstetter WL. Tumors of the diaphragm [review]. Thorac Surg Clin 2009; 19(4):521–9.

Pulmonary Assessment for General Thoracic Surgery

Farzaneh Banki, MD

KEYWORDS

• Pulmonary assessment • General thoracic surgery
• Postoperative pulmonary complications • Pulmonary resection

Preoperative pulmonary assessment is an essential step in the selection and the management of patients who are candidates for thoracic procedures. Despite advances in anesthesia, including the use of epidural analgesics, and advances in surgical techniques and perioperative care, postoperative pulmonary complications remain the leading cause of morbidity and mortality in thoracic surgery. A postoperative pulmonary complication is defined as a pulmonary abnormality that produces identifiable disease or dysfunction that is clinically significant and adversely affects patients' postoperative course. The definition of postoperative pulmonary complications following thoracic procedures may be variable, but includes those in **Box 1**. Complications, such as bronchopleural fistula and hemothorax, requiring chest tube placement or reoperation are considered surgical complications.

Pulmonary complications, particularly in patients undergoing lung resection, prolong hospital stay and cost, are associated with increased operative mortality, and predict long-term disability.[1,2] The incidence of postoperative pulmonary complications after thoracotomy and lung resection is about 30% and is not only related to the removal of lung tissue but is also caused by alterations in chest wall mechanics caused by the thoracotomy itself.[3,4] All spirometric measurements fall precipitously immediately following surgery and do not return to normal until 6 to 8 weeks postoperatively.[5] Postoperative pulmonary dysfunction appears to be less common after video-assisted thoracoscopic surgery (VATS) procedures than after thoracotomy. In a nonrandomized comparison of subjects who had a lobectomy by a thoracotomy versus VATS, postoperative PaO2, O2 saturation, peak flow rates, forced expiratory volume in 1 second (FEV1), and forced vital capacity (FVC) on both postoperative days 7 and 14 were better in subjects who had undergone the VATS procedure.[6] Following VATS lobectomy, there was less impairment of pulmonary function and a better 6-minute walk test.[7] VATS lobectomy leads to only a 15% loss in vital capacity

Department of Cardiothoracic and Vascular Surgery, The University of Texas Medical School at Houston, 6400 Fannin Street, Suite 2850, Houston, TX 77030, USA
E-mail address: farzaneh.banki@uth.tmc.edu

Surg Clin N Am 90 (2010) 969–984
doi:10.1016/j.suc.2010.07.001
0039-6109/10/$ – see front matter © 2010 Elsevier Inc. All rights reserved.

surgical.theclinics.com

Box 1
Definition of postoperative pulmonary complications within 30 days of surgery

1. Acute CO2 retention (partial pressure of arterial CO2 45 mm Hg)

2. Prolonged mechanical ventilation greater than 24 hours

3. Reintubation for respiratory failure

4. Adult respiratory distress syndrome

5. Pneumonia, temperature greater than 38°C, purulent sputum, and infiltrate on chest radiograph

6. Pulmonary embolism (high probability ventilation/perfusion scan or diagnostic pulmonary angiogram)

7. Lobar atelectasis requiring bronchoscopy

8. Need for O2 at the time of discharge

---

and FEV1; whereas, open thoracotomy leads to losses of 23% and 29%, respectively.[8]

Similarly in patients who undergo esophagectomy, postoperative pulmonary complications occur in 15% to 40% of patients.[9,10] The reasons for this high risk in patients who undergo esophagectomy is multifactorial and includes surgical entry into 2 separate body cavities, disruption of bronchial innervation and lymphatic circulation, dysfunction of the diaphragm, poor airway protection secondary to recurrent laryngeal nerve injury, and uncoordinated deglutition. These complications may be reduced in patients who undergo minimally invasive esophagectomy. In a series of 222 subjects undergoing minimally invasive esophagectomy, Luketich and colleagues[11] reported pneumonia in 7.7%, pleural effusion requiring drainage in 6.3%, and atelectasis requiring bronchoscopy in 4.5%.

Despite improvements in anesthesia and preoperative and postoperative care, pulmonary complications remain common following thoracic procedures. Therefore, a comprehensive preoperative pulmonary assessment and careful selection of patients for general thoracic procedures, particularly in patients who undergo pulmonary resection or esophagectomy, is necessary to assess the operative risk, to decrease the risk of postoperative complications, and to achieve better outcomes.

HISTORY AND PHYSICAL EXAMINATION

A careful history that focuses on eliciting respiratory complaints, such as fever, cough, dyspnea, chest pain, exercise intolerance, and excessive sputum production, may assist clinicians in identifying conditions (eg, the presence of an intrabronchial lesion, pleural effusion, interstitial lung disease, chronic obstructive pulmonary disease) and social habits, such as smoking, that could increase the risk for postoperative pulmonary complications. Preoperative dyspnea scores, for instance, have been shown to correlate well with postoperative pulmonary complications in several studies.[12]

Although generally insensitive as a screening test, a thorough history and physical examination are inexpensive and provide an opportunity to consolidate information about patients and the planned operation, and to recommend a course of action for modifying risks in selected groups of patients, especially those with preexisting chronic obstructive pulmonary disease and smokers.

SPIROMETRY

Spirometry has been used to predict the risk of complications after lung resection for more than 50 years. In 1955, Gaensler and colleagues[13] assessed the role of pulmonary insufficiency in mortality following surgery for pulmonary tuberculosis and included the use of spirometry. They were the first to show that patients undergoing lung resection surgery, who had a maximum voluntary ventilation of less than 50% and a forced vital capacity less than 70%, had a 40% postoperative mortality. Spirometry is still considered to be the mainstay for the selection of candidates for lung resection.[1,14,15] Poor respiratory function is a concern because of the risk of perioperative mortality, the possibility of postoperative pulmonary complications, long-term disability, and poor quality of life secondary to respiratory insufficiency. These risks are related to preexisting pulmonary dysfunction and the extent of the planned surgery.

FORCED EXPIRATORY VOLUME IN 1 SECOND

Data from more than 2000 subjects in 3 large series in the 1970s have shown that a mortality rate of less than 5% should be expected if the preoperative FEV1 is greater than 1.5 L for a lobectomy and greater than 2 L for a pneumonectomy.[2,16,17]

In 1971, Boushy and colleagues[16] found an FEV1 less than 2 L and FEV1/FVC less than 50% to be poor prognostic signs in patients older than 60 years of age undergoing pulmonary resection for lung cancer. Lockwood[18] showed that FEV1 less than 1.2 L or less than 35% of FVC indicate a high risk for lung resection. Miller and colleagues[19] studied complications in 500 subjects undergoing lung resection and correlated the postoperative complications with preoperative spirometric indexes and type of surgery performed. Based on the results of their study, the recommended requirements for a pneumonectomy were FEV1 greater than 2 L; for a lobectomy, FEV1 greater than1 L; and for a segmentectomy or wedge resection, FEV1 greater than 0.6 L. Using these criteria, the reported mortality rate was 0.2% for segmental or wedge resection, 0.0% for lobectomy, and 4.4% for pneumonectomy. A retrospective study of 236 subjects by Stephan and colleagues[20] showed that the incidence of postoperative pulmonary complications in subjects with FEV1 values less than 2 L was 40% versus 19% for those with FEV1 greater than 2 L.

Other authors have performed pulmonary resection in patients with marginal FEV1. Linden and colleagues,[21] in a study of 100 subjects who underwent lung resection for cancer, assessed the morbidity, mortality, and feasibility of pulmonary resection in subjects with preoperative FEV1 less than 35% of the predicted value and an average preoperative FEV1 of 26% of the predicted value. There was 1 death. Thirty-six percent of the subjects had 1 or more complications. A total of 22% of the subjects had prolonged air leaks requiring a chest tube for more than 7 days, 4 subjects had pneumonia, 1 subject left the hospital ventilator dependent, 3 additional subjects required intubation for more than 48 hours, and 11 subjects were discharged with a new oxygen requirement. Male gender ($P = .003$), preoperative oxygen dependence ($P = .03$), and pack-year history ($P = .006$) were associated with a higher overall incidence of complications; whereas, age and preoperative percentage of the predicted FEV1 did not correlate with the overall incidence of complications in their study. They concluded that in a large academic center, with the use of minimally invasive surgical techniques, intensive pulmonary care, and advanced anesthetic techniques, it is feasible to perform pulmonary resection in patients with low preoperative FEV1 with a low mortality and low incidence of ventilator dependence, but an extended hospital stay and a high incidence of prolonged air leak should be expected, especially in patients with preoperative FEV1 less than or equal to 20% of the predicted value.

DIFFUSING CAPACITY FOR CARBON MONOXIDE OR GAS TRANSFER FACTOR

Diffusing capacity for carbon monoxide or gas transfer factor (DLCO) or gas transfer factor is a surrogate measurement of oxygen uptake capacity of the lungs and reflects the alveolar membrane integrity and pulmonary capillary blood flow in patients' lungs. Abnormal DLCO values may represent a defect in gas exchange, which could be at the level of the alveolar epithelium, the pulmonary vasculature, or the interstitium of the lung.

DLCO percentage has been considered as an independent predictor of postoperative pulmonary complication after major lung resection. Ferguson and colleagues[22] reported that when DLCO was less than 60%, the rate of pulmonary complications was 45%, and when DLCO was greater than 100%, the rate of pulmonary complications was only 11%. It is possible that some patients may have good spirometric values but a very low DLCO because of diffuse interstitial lung disease. These patients should be assessed more carefully. Wang and colleagues[23] assessed the utility of DLCO percentage in prediction of postoperative pulmonary complications, and the effect of such complication in 40 subjects who underwent lung resection. They showed that DLCO predicted pulmonary complication after major lung resection. Further, it was shown that the absence of an increase in DLCO with exercise was 78% sensitive and 100% specific for predicting postoperative pulmonary complications.[24]

QUANTITATIVE VENTILATION PERFUSION SCAN

Quantitative ventilation perfusion scan is a useful tool to predict postoperative pulmonary function after lung resection.[25] This test is particularly important in patients with marginal pulmonary reserve.

The estimation of the postoperative FEV1 (FEV1-ppo) as percent predicted in patients who undergo pneumonectomy can be calculated by obtaining preoperative FEV1 and the quantitative ventilation perfusion scan to obtain the fraction of the total lung perfusion present in the lung to be resected, using the following formula:[26]

% FEV1-ppo = FEV1-pre × (1– fraction of total perfusion resected lung)

For pneumonectomy there is a strong correlation between the postoperative FEV1 expressed as percent predicted and calculated from the quantitative lung perfusion scans, and the actual values.[2,17,26–28]

Estimated postoperative FEV1 (FEV1-ppo) expressed as percent after lobectomy can be calculated by different arithmetic calculations. NaKahara and colleagues[29] include the obstructed segment as part of the calculation to measure the FEV1-ppo, using the following formula:

FEV1-ppo = FEV1-pre × [(19 – a) – b]/(19-a)

In this formula, a represents the number of obstructed segments to be resected, and b represents the number of unobstructed segments to be resected. The segments in each lung are as follows: right upper lobe 3; middle lobe 2; right lower lobe 5; left upper lobe 3; lingula 2; left lower lobe 4, for a total of 19 segments. The same calculations can be applied to the postoperative DLCO (DLCO -ppo).

The simplest formula assumes equal distribution of lung function between 19 lobar segments. (10 on the right and 9 on the left) and approximately 5% function for each segment. The FEV1 -ppo estimated as follows:

%FEV1-ppo = preoperative FEV1 × (no. residual segments)/(no. initial segments)

For lobectomy, there is a strong correlation between the postoperative FEV1 expressed as percent predicted and the actual values when the calculation is made depending upon the number of segments to be removed at lobectomy.[17,30]

Traditionally, a predicted postoperative FEV1 (FEV1-ppo) of 0.8 L (based on perfusion scintigraphy) was the minimal accepted FEV1 for patients undergoing resection.[1,31,32] However, 0.8 L as a single value cannot be used to discriminate between patients of different age, size, sexe, and level of cardiovascular fitness.

There is substantial evidence that the perioperative risks of resection are related to the absolute predicted postoperative FEV1,[15,31,33,34] and the postoperative FEV1 expressed as percent predicted.[1,15,34,35]

EXERCISE TESTING

An inverse relationship between exercise capacity and postoperative complications has been demonstrated in several studies using both simple exercise tests, such as 6-minute walks, stair climbs, and formal cardiopulmonary exercise test.[1,15,36–40]

Stair climbing is an easy and rapid way to assess exercise capacity and cardiopulmonary reserve. In 1968, Van Nostrand and colleagues[41] published a retrospective review of subjects who underwent pneumonectomy and had performed a preoperative stair climb. These investigators noted a mortality rate of 11% among subjects who were able to climb more than 2 flights of stairs. However, in subjects who were unable to climb 2 flights of stairs, 2 out of 4 (50%) died. Olsen and colleagues,[39] in a retrospective review of 84 subjects who underwent lung resection and had preoperative stair climb before lung resection, showed that subjects unable to climb 3 flights of stairs had a higher number of postoperative complications, longer intubations, and longer postoperative lengths of stay compared with those subjects able to climb 3 flights of stairs. Holden and colleagues,[36] in a study of 23 high-risk subjects with FEV1 less than 1.6 L who underwent lung resection, showed a 6-minute walk distance of greater than 1000 ft and a stair climb of greater than 44 steps were predictive of successful surgical outcome. Brunelli and colleagues[42–45] found that the results of a stair-climbing test accurately predicted postoperative pulmonary complications in subjects who had an FEV1 of less than 40% of the predicted value and in those more than 70 years of age.

MAXIMUM OXYGEN CONSUMPTION

Although pulmonary function tests initially identify patients at high risk for pulmonary resection, in patients with marginal pulmonary function, such as FEV1 less than 60% and DLCO less than 60% of the predicted value, or FEV1-ppo less than 40% and DLCO –ppo less than 40%, further diagnostic modalities are required to assess the surgical risk and the postoperative pulmonary complications. One useful and simple diagnostic modality is cardiopulmonary exercise testing with measurement of the maximum oxygen consumption (VO2 max), which provides a tool for physiologic assessment in patients who are candidates for lung surgery.

VO2 in the lungs is representative of VO2 at the cellular level. With an increase in the cellular respiration from exercise, there is a predictable increase in VO2, which is related to age, sex, weight, and type of work performed. A formula for estimating VO2 reported by Wasserman and Whipp[46] is as follows:

Predicted VO2 = 5.8 × weight in kg + 151 + 10.1W, where *W* is workload

VO2 increases with exercise until a point at which a plateau is reached and a further increase in work does not result in a continued rise in VO2, this level represents the VO2 max.[47] Increasingly, cardiopulmonary exercise testing is being used because it provides the best index of functional capacity and VO2 max, as well as estimating both cardiac and pulmonary reserves not available from other modalities. Cardiopulmonary exercise testing permits the detection of clinically occult heart disease and provides a more reliable estimate of functional capacity postoperatively compared with pulmonary function testing. Further, VO2 max is an independent predictor of operative risk in patients who undergo pulmonary resection. Both pulmonary function tests and VO2 max studies are complementary and help in the assessment of surgical risk; this is particularly valuable for borderline patients so that the opportunity for curative resection is not denied.[48] Of the screening exercise tests available, the shuttle walk test[49] is more reproducible[49–51] and has a higher correlation with VO2 max estimated by formal exercise testing than the 6-minute walk test.[52,53]

The percent predicted maximum oxygen consumption accurately predicted postoperative pulmonary complications in a series of subjects undergoing thoracic surgery for lung cancer.[54] A preoperative VO2 max of more than 15 mL/kg/min is associated with no appreciable increase in perioperative mortality and pulmonary complications; whereas, patients with VO2 max of less than 10 mL/kg/min are not candidates for pulmonary resection because of the high risk of postoperative pulmonary complications.[1,33,52,55–58] Patients with VO2 max between 10 to 15 mL/kg/min should be assessed individually by considering the functional status and other risk factors.

Arterial Blood Gas and Oxygen Saturation at Rest

Arterial blood gas demonstration of hypercapnia of $PaCo_2$ greater than 45 torr and hypoxemia of PaO_2 less than 55 torr had been considered in the past as indices of high risk for postoperative complication and contraindications for thoracic surgery.[12,59–61] These values are now recognized to be only relative contraindications. Recent studies have shown that hypercapnia is not per se predictive of complications after resection, particularly if patients who are able to exercise adequately.[15,57,62,63] However, such patients are often precluded because of other adverse factors on pulmonary function testing. Ninan and colleagues[37] found that there was a higher risk of postoperative complications among patients who either had oxygen saturation (SaO_2) on air at rest of less than 90% or desaturated by greater than 4% from baseline during exercise.

THRESHOLDS FOR POSTOPERATIVE PREDICTED VALUES

In 2001, the British Thoracic Society and the Society of Cardiothoracic Surgeons of Great Britain published guidelines for selection of patients with lung cancer for surgery. A summary of the guidelines for the pulmonary assessment is presented in **Box 2**.[64]

Further, in 2003 the American College of Chest Physicians (ACCP) published an evidence-based guideline for the diagnosis and management of patients with lung cancer that included a series of recommendations regarding the use of preoperative physiologic evaluation (**Box 3**).[65]

A range of values for postoperative FEV1 between 34% and 45% of the predicted value has been recommended as the lower limit of operability.[62,66] For FEV1, a large study by Markos and colleagues[1] recommended a figure of 40%. Similarly, for the DLCO a figure of 40% has been recommended.[1,34] The study by Pierce and colleagues[34] supports the conclusion that both FEV1 and DLCO are independent prognostic factors.

Box 2
Risk assessment for patients who undergo pulmonary resection

1. No further respiratory function tests are required for a lobectomy if the postbronchodilator FEV1 is greater than 1.5 L and for a pneumonectomy if the postbronchodilator FEV1 is greater than 2.0 L, provided that there is no evidence of interstitial lung disease or unexpected disability caused by shortness of breath.

2. All patients not clearly operable on the basis of FEV1 should have: (1) estimation of DLCO, (2) measurement of oxygen saturation on air at rest, and (3) a quantitative isotope perfusion scan if a pneumonectomy is being considered.

3. The estimated postoperative FEV1 expressed as percent predicted and the estimated postoperative DLCO expressed as percent predicted should be calculated using either the lung scan for pneumonectomy or an anatomic equation for lobectomy, taking into account whether the segments to be removed are ventilated or obstructed.

4. Estimated postoperative FEV1 less than 40% of the predicted value and estimated postoperative DLCO less than 40% of the predicted value is considered high risk and patients should be referred for exercise testing.

5. Best distance on 2 shuttle walk tests of less than 25 shuttles (250 m) or desaturation during the test of more than 4% SaO2 is considered high risk for surgery.

   Other patients should be referred for a formal cardiopulmonary exercise test. A VO2 max of less than 15 mL/kg/min indicates that patients are a high risk for surgery.

Data from BTS guidelines: guidelines on the selection of patients with lung cancer for surgery. Thorax 2001;56:89–108; with permission.

The summary of the previously mentioned studies shows that if FEV1 values of greater than 2 L or greater than 60% of the predicted value, and DLCO values of greater than 60% of the predicted value are obtained, patients are at low risk for complications and can undergo pulmonary resection, including pneumonectomy, without further testing. If the previously mentioned requirements are not met, patients need further evaluation.[47] The acceptable threshold values for preoperative FEV1 and DLCO are variable and range between 60% to 80%, but the FEV1-ppo of 40% and DLCO-ppo of 40% seems to be a universally acceptable threshold for pulmonary

---

Box 3
Preoperative physiologic assessment of patients with lung cancer undergoing lung resection (The ACCP-published, evidence-based guidelines)

1. Spirometry should be performed in patients being considered for resection, if FEV1 is greater than 80% of the predicted value or greater than 2 L, patients are suitable for pneumonectomy without further evaluation; if the FEV1 is greater than 1.5 L, patients are suitable for lobectomy without further evaluation.

2. Patients with evidence of interstitial lung disease on radiographs or dyspnea on exertion should have DLCO measured even though FEV1 may be adequate.

3. If either the FEV1 or DLCO is less than 80% of the predicted value, postoperative lung function should be predicted on the basis of additional testing.

4. Exercise testing is indicated preoperatively in patients with a percent ppo FEV1 less than 40% of the predicted value or percent ppo DLCO less than 40% of the predicted value.

Data from Beckles MA, Spiro SG, Colice GL, et al. The physiologic evaluation of patients with lung cancer being considered for resectional surgery. Chest 2003;123:105S–14S.

resection by the majority of the studies. A simple algorithm for the preoperative evaluation before pulmonary resection is shown in **Fig. 1**.

SCORING SYSTEMS

Several scoring systems have been developed in an attempt to provide a comprehensive approach to the preoperative assessment of patients with pulmonary disease undergoing thoracic surgery, including the Physiologic and Operative Severity Score for Enumeration of Mortality and Morbidity (POSSUM).[67] The POSSUM data set was developed by Copeland and colleagues[68] in 1991. From 35 possible risk factors for adverse outcome after an operation, 12 preoperative factors were found to be independently predictive and were included in the final POSSUM data set. Brunelli and colleagues[69] prospectively applied the POSSUM scoring system to 250 consecutive subjects who underwent pulmonary resection for lung cancer, including 160 lobectomies and 54 pneumonectomies, to evaluate its ability to predict postoperative complications, including pulmonary complications. The preoperative factors included respiratory status, cardiac status, and the hemoglobin level, among others. Logistic regression analysis showed POSSUM was predictive of postoperative complications, showing no significant difference between predicted and observed postoperative pulmonary complications in patients who undergo lung resection.

Cardiopulmonary Risk Index (CPRI) is a multifactorial index intended to predict postoperative outcome after thoracic surgery. It combines cardiac and pulmonary information into one parameter that ranges from 1 to 10, with 10 being the worst. A CPRI greater than or equal to 4 has been advocated as a reliable predictor of postoperative pulmonary and cardiac complications. In a prospective study, Melendez and colleagues[70] evaluated the predictive value of CPRI in 180 subjects who underwent pulmonary resection. Postoperative complications, among others, included pneumonia, atelectasis, respiratory failure requiring therapy, or death occurring 30 days of surgery. They found that a CPRI greater than or equal to 4 to be a moderate predictor of outcome for subjects undergoing pneumonectomy (n = 19). They concluded that the preoperative CPRI and its components were inadequate predictors of medical complications after thoracic surgery in a general population, but in the subgroup of subjects undergoing pneumonectomy, the index may be of some value.

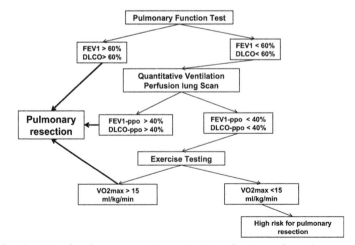

Fig. 1. The algorithm for the preoperative evaluation of patients for pulmonary resection.

Furgeson and colleagues,[71] in a retrospective review of 400 subjects who underwent pulmonary resection for lung cancer, developed a simplified scoring system, called Expiratory Volume Age Diffusion capacity (EVAD). This score is based on 3 predictive covariates: age, spirometry, and diffusing capacity. This system was then evaluated against the POSSUM and CPRI systems. Receiver operating characteristic analysis demonstrated the EVAD system to be equivalent to or better than CPRI and POSSUM for all complication categories. They concluded that a simple scoring system (EVAD) that uses pulmonary function test data and patient age is easier to use and at least as accurate as other scoring systems currently in use for predicting the likelihood of complications after major lung resection.

MODIFIABLE RISK FACTORS
Pulmonary Rehabilitation

Pulmonary rehabilitation has been best studied in patients with chronic obstructive pulmonary disease. Regardless of the severity of chronic obstructive pulmonary disease, pulmonary rehabilitation has been shown to be effective in reducing symptoms, increasing daily activity, and minimizing exacerbations.[72,73] The role of pulmonary rehabilitation in a preoperative setting has been largely explored in patients with pulmonary emphysema undergoing lung volume resection surgery. In the National Emphysema Treatment Trial, pulmonary rehabilitation was considered an inclusion criterion before randomization to undergo surgery.[74] The value of pulmonary rehabilitation in patient screening, exercise testing, and individualized exercise prescription has been established, and preoperative pulmonary rehabilitation has been shown to lead to a significant improvement in exercise capacity, dyspnea, and health-related quality of life.[75–77] The impact of pulmonary rehabilitation on postoperative morbidity and mortality after pulmonary resection is not well established, but a few studies have suggested benefits for pulmonary rehabilitation before pulmonary resection in patients with lung cancer. Sekine and colleagues,[78] in a study of 22 subjects with lung cancer who received pulmonary rehabilitation, reported that the hospital stay was shorter and postoperative FEV1 values were improved in these subjects compared with control subjects with higher preoperative FEV1 values that did not undergo preoperative pulmonary rehabilitation. Pulmonary rehabilitation included exercise training, nutrition education, medication adjustment, training in breathing techniques, and group therapy.

Bobbio and colleagues[79] studied the impact of short-term preoperative pulmonary rehabilitation on exercise capacity in subjects with chronic obstructive pulmonary disease undergoing lobectomy for non-small cell lung cancer. The maximal oxygen consumption by cardio-pulmonary exercise testing was evaluated and when VO2 max was less than or equal to 15 mL/kg/min, a pulmonary rehabilitation program lasting 4 weeks was considered. Twelve subjects completed the preoperative rehabilitation program and underwent a new functional evaluation before surgery. Preparation for intervention for all subjects included the cessation of smoking and optimization of pharmacologic treatment. Bronchodilators were prescribed; whereas, steroids were not introduced. The pulmonary rehabilitation program consisted of a 1.5-hour hospital appointment 5 days a week for 4 weeks. During the first session subjects were taught controlled breathing and cough techniques and were instructed on incentive spirometry exercises. They were asked to repeat the exercises twice daily at home. The peripheral muscle exercise training program consisted of aerobic work on a leg cycle ergometer. Each training session consisted of a 5-minute warm-up at 30% of maximal work rate, followed by 30 minutes at 50% of maximal work rate, ending with a 5-minute cool-down. Workloads were calculated from the work rate obtained during the cardiopulmonary exercise testing and were then progressively increased weekly up to 80% of the maximal work rate. At the end of cycling, subjects underwent muscle stretching for 10 minutes and the session was then completed with upper-extremity and trunk-muscle conditioning free-weight exercises. Trained medical and physical therapist staff supervised subjects during the whole session.

On completion of pulmonary rehabilitation, pulmonary function tests and lung diffusion capacity were unchanged; whereas, the exercise performance was found to have significantly improved. The mean increase in maximal oxygen consumption proved to be at 2.8 mL/kg/min (P<.01). They concluded that preoperative pulmonary rehabilitation could improve the exercise capacity of patients with chronic obstructive pulmonary disease who are candidates for lung resection for non-small cell lung cancer.

Cigarette Use

Cigarette smoking is a significant and preventable cause of morbidity and mortality in the United States[80] and is associated with increased risk of postoperative pulmonary complications in thoracic surgery. Nagakawa and colleagues,[81] in a study of 288 subjects who underwent pulmonary surgery, examined the relationship between the duration of the preoperative smoke-free period and the development of postoperative pulmonary complications to determine the optimal timing for cessation of smoking before surgery. Study subjects were classified into 4 groups based on their smoking status. A current smoker was defined as one who smoked within 2 weeks before the operation. Recent smokers and ex-smokers were defined as those whose duration of abstinence from smoking was 2 to 4 weeks and more than 4 weeks before the operation, respectively. A never-smoker was defined as one who had never smoked. The incidence of postoperative pulmonary complications among the current smokers and recent smokers was 43.6% and 53.8%, respectively, and each was higher than that among those who had never smoked (23.9%; P<.05). The incidence of postoperative pulmonary complications gradually decreased in subjects whose smoke-free period was 5 to 8 weeks or longer. After controlling for sex, age, results of pulmonary function tests, and duration of surgery, the odds ratios for postoperative pulmonary complications developing in current smokers, recent smokers, and ex-smokers in comparison with never-smokers were 2.09, 2.44, and 1.03, respectively. They concluded that to reduce the incidence of postoperative pulmonary complications subjects needed to stop smoking for at least 4 weeks before pulmonary surgery. Vaporciyan and colleagues,[82] in a retrospective review of 261 subjects who underwent pneumonectomy for malignant disease showed that only the timing of smoking cessation (1 month or less before operation) was a significant predictor of major pulmonary complications, including pneumonia and adult respiratory distress syndrome. Age, side of pneumonectomy, and the use of preoperative chemotherapy or combined chemotherapy and radiation therapy were not significant predictor factors for major pulmonary complications. In a study of 311 subjects operated for non-small cell lung cancer, Sardari Nia and colleagues[83] showed that current smoking was an independent predictor of poor prognosis, and nonsmokers, former smokers, and recent quitters had a significant better prognosis compared with current smokers. They concluded that smoking cessation is beneficial for patients with lung cancer at any point before lung operation; whereas, smoking up to the time of operation is associated with a worse prognosis.

PULMONARY ASSESSMENT BEFORE ESOPHAGECTOMY

Pulmonary complications, such as pneumonia and respiratory insufficiency, are among the most frequent complications after esophagectomy. The risk of pulmonary complications after esophagectomy is higher than any other operation, including major lung resection. Therefore, preoperative pulmonary assessment is important to identify the patients who are at the highest risk.

A high incidence of pulmonary complications after esophagectomy has been recognized for decades, and a variety of intraoperative and postoperative techniques have been used in an attempt to reduce the frequency of this problem, including incentive spirometry, intermittent positive-pressure breathing, and chest physiotherapy.[84,85] Attempts to develop systems for predicting which patients are at increased risk to develop pulmonary complications have been only partially successful. In addition, many studies identify factors (intraoperative blood loss, use of epidural analgesia, use of bronchoscopy postoperative to clear secretions, tumor stage, and duration of the operation) that cannot be used to preoperatively predict the risk of complications.[85,86] A multicenter prospective study of 1777 subjects undergoing esophagectomy reported by Bailey and colleagues[87] found a 21% incidence of pneumonia and a 16% incidence of respiratory failure. Preoperative factors associated with postoperative complications, among others, were dyspnea, chronic obstructive pulmonary disease, and decreased functional status. In a trial of 220 subjects with adenocarcinoma of the mid-to-distal esophagus or the gastric cardiac involving the distal esophagus randomized to undergo esophagectomy via a transhiatal approach versus a transthoracic approach, Hulscher and colleagues[88] showed a lower incidence of postoperative pulmonary complications (27% vs 57%, respectively; $P<.001$) with the transhiatal approach.

Pulmonary function has long been known to be associated with pulmonary complications after esophagectomy. Fan and colleagues[89] suggested that a preoperative peak expiratory flow rate of less than 65% of predicted correlated well with the incidence of pulmonary complications. However, preoperative peak expiratory flow rate had less predictive value than other variables, including age, albumin level, and arterial oxygen tension. Nagawa and colleagues[86] reported a significant difference in vital capacity between subjects who developed pulmonary complications and those who did not. However, the mean vital capacity of subjects who developed pulmonary complications was still 91.8% of the predicted value, which is normal.

Ferguson and colleagues,[90] in a review of 292 subjects who underwent esophagectomy for cancer, identified factors associated with the development of pulmonary complications and developed a scoring system to predict risk. The scoring system included age, spirometry, and performance. Pulmonary complication happened in 78 (26.7%) of the subjects. Multivariable analysis identified the important covariates to be patient age, FEV1 percentage, and performance status. These 3 covariates were combined into a scoring system. The accuracy of this scoring system in predicting postoperative pulmonary complications was 65.4%. Avenado and colleagues,[91] in a study of 61 subjects who underwent esophagectomy for esophageal cancer, showed that pneumonia was the most common clinically important complication, with 19.7% of subjects requiring prolonged ventilatory support. Significant risk factors identified included impaired pulmonary function, especially for subjects with FEV1 less than 65% of the predicted value.

SUMMARY

Preoperative pulmonary assessment in patients who present for consideration of thoracic surgery is a crucial part of their evaluation, and knowledge of different tests and parameters that can predict the risk of postoperative pulmonary complications and mortality is essential. For pulmonary resection, a combination of FEV1 and

Banki

DLCO remain the most useful studies. Ventilation perfusion scans are particularly important in patients with a marginal pulmonary function test and can be used to estimate postoperative FEV1 and DLCO. V02 max is an indicator of cardiopulmonary status and values greater than 15 cc/kg/min are adequate for pulmonary resection.

In patients who undergo esophagectomy, the risk of postoperative pulmonary complications is high, and careful selection of patients is crucial to improve outcomes. Patients with FEV1 greater than 65% of the predicted value appear to have adequate pulmonary reserve for an esophagectomy.

No single parameter is predictive of postoperative complications or mortality in patients who undergo a thoracic procedure. Therefore, patients should not be denied for surgical resection based on any single abnormal test or parameter. A comprehensive assessment of the functional status, exercise tolerance, and pulmonary function should be performed before surgery to select the patients appropriately, predict the risk of postoperative complications, and achieve better outcomes.

REFERENCES

1. Markos J, Mullan BP, Hillman DR, et al. Preoperative assessment as a predictor of mortality and morbidity after lung resection. Am Rev Respir Dis 1989;139:902–10.
2. Miller JI Jr. Physiologic evaluation of pulmonary function in the candidate for lung resection. J Thorac Cardiovasc Surg 1993;105:347–51 [discussion: 351–2].
3. Hazelrigg SR, Landreneau RJ, Boley TM, et al. The effect of muscle-sparing versus standard posterolateral thoracotomy on pulmonary function, muscle strength, and postoperative pain. J Thorac Cardiovasc Surg 1991;101:394–400 [discussion: 400–1].
4. Busch E, Verazin G, Antkowiak JG, et al. Pulmonary complications in patients undergoing thoracotomy for lung carcinoma. Chest 1994;105:760–6.
5. Bastin R, Moraine JJ, Bardocsky G, et al. Incentive spirometry performance. A reliable indicator of pulmonary function in the early postoperative period after lobectomy? Chest 1997;111:559–63.
6. Nakata M, Saeki H, Yokoyama N, et al. Pulmonary function after lobectomy: video-assisted thoracic surgery versus thoracotomy. Ann Thorac Surg 2000;70:938–41.
7. Nomori H, Ohtsuka T, Horio H, et al. Difference in the impairment of vital capacity and 6-minute walking after a lobectomy performed by thoracoscopic surgery, an anterior limited thoracotomy, an anteroaxillary thoracotomy, and a posterolateral thoracotomy. Surg Today 2003;33:7–12.
8. Kaseda S, Aoki T, Hangai N, Shimizu K. Better pulmonary function and prognosis with video-assisted thoracic surgery than with thoracotomy. Ann Thorac Surg 2000;70:1644–6.
9. Law SY, Fok M, Wong J. Risk analysis in resection of squamous cell carcinoma of the esophagus. World J Surg 1994;18:339–46.
10. Gockel I, Exner C, Junginger T. Morbidity and mortality after esophagectomy for esophageal carcinoma: a risk analysis. World J Surg Oncol 2005;3:37.
11. Luketich JD, Alvelo-Rivera M, Buenaventura PO, et al. Minimally invasive esophagectomy: outcomes in 222 patients. Ann Surg 2003;238:486–94 [discussion: 494–5].
12. Milledge JS, Nunn JF. Criteria of fitness for anaesthesia in patients with chronic obstructive lung disease. Br Med J 1975;3:670–3.
13. Gaensler EA, Cugell DW, Lindgren I, et al. The role of pulmonary insufficiency in mortality and invalidism following surgery for pulmonary tuberculosis. J Thorac Surg 1955;29:163–87.

14. Ferguson MK, Reeder LB, Mick R. Optimizing selection of patients for major lung resection. J Thorac Cardiovasc Surg 1995;109:275–81 [discussion: 281–3].

15. Kearney DJ, Lee TH, Reilly JJ, et al. Assessment of operative risk in patients undergoing lung resection. Importance of predicted pulmonary function. Chest 1994;105:753–9.

16. Boushy SF, Billig DM, North LB, Helgason AH. Clinical course related to preoperative and postoperative pulmonary function in patients with bronchogenic carcinoma. Chest 1971;59:383–91.

17. Wernly JA, DeMeester TR, Kirchner PT, et al. Clinical value of quantitative ventilation-perfusion lung scans in the surgical management of bronchogenic carcinoma. J Thorac Cardiovasc Surg 1980;80:535–43.

18. Lockwood P. Lung function test results and the risk of post-thoracotomy complications. Respiration 1973;30:529–42.

19. Miller JI, Grossman GD, Hatcher CR. Pulmonary function test criteria for operability and pulmonary resection. Surg Gynecol Obstet 1981;153:893–5.

20. Stephan F, Boucheseiche S, Hollande J, et al. Pulmonary complications following lung resection: a comprehensive analysis of incidence and possible risk factors. Chest 2000;118:1263–70.

21. Linden PA, Bueno R, Colson YL, et al. Lung resection in patients with preoperative FEV1 < 35% predicted. Chest 2005;127:1984–90.

22. Ferguson MK, Little L, Rizzo L, et al. Diffusing capacity predicts morbidity and mortality after pulmonary resection. J Thorac Cardiovasc Surg 1988;96:894–900.

23. Wang J, Olak J, Ultmann RE, Ferguson MK. Assessment of pulmonary complications after lung resection. Ann Thorac Surg 1999;67:1444–7.

24. Wang JS. Pulmonary function tests in preoperative pulmonary evaluation. Respir Med 2004;98:598–605.

25. Olsen GN, Weiman DS, Bolton JW, et al. Submaximal invasive exercise testing and quantitative lung scanning in the evaluation for tolerance of lung resection. Chest 1989;95:267–73.

26. Corris PA, Ellis DA, Hawkins T, Gibson GJ. Use of radionuclide scanning in the preoperative estimation of pulmonary function after pneumonectomy. Thorax 1987;42:285–91.

27. Boysen PG, Harris JO, Block AJ, Olsen GN. Prospective evaluation for pneumonectomy using perfusion scanning: follow-up beyond one year. Chest 1981;80:163–6.

28. Ellis DA, Hawkins T, Gibson GJ, Nariman S. Role of lung scanning in assessing the resectability of bronchial carcinoma. Thorax 1983;38:261–6.

29. Nakahara K, Monden Y, Ohno K, et al. 1985: a method for predicting postoperative lung function and its relation to postoperative complications in patients with lung cancer. 1992 update. Ann Thorac Surg 1992;54:1016–7.

30. Zeiher BG, Gross TJ, Kern JA, et al. Predicting postoperative pulmonary function in patients undergoing lung resection. Chest 1995;108:68–72.

31. Olsen GN, Block AJ, Swenson EW, et al. Pulmonary function evaluation of the lung resection candidate: a prospective study. Am Rev Respir Dis 1975;111:379–87.

32. Boysen PG, Block AJ, Moulder PV. Relationship between preoperative pulmonary function tests and complications after thoracotomy. Surg Gynecol Obstet 1981;152:813–5.

33. Pate P, Tenholder MF, Griffin JP, et al. Preoperative assessment of the high-risk patient for lung resection. Ann Thorac Surg 1996;61:1494–500.

34. Pierce RJ, Copland JM, Sharpe K, Barter CE. Preoperative risk evaluation for lung cancer resection: predicted postoperative product as a predictor of surgical mortality. Am J Respir Crit Care Med 1994;150:947–55.

35. Brunelli A, Fianchini A. Predicted postoperative FEV1 and complications in lung resection candidates. Chest 1997;111:1145–6.
36. Holden DA, Rice TW, Stelmach K, Meeker DP. Exercise testing, 6-min walk, and stair climb in the evaluation of patients at high risk for pulmonary resection. Chest 1992;102:1774–9.
37. Ninan M, Sommers KE, Landreneau RJ, et al. Standardized exercise oximetry predicts postpneumonectomy outcome. Ann Thorac Surg 1997;64:328–32 [discussion: 332–3].
38. Rao V, Todd TR, Kuus A, et al. Exercise oximetry versus spirometry in the assessment of risk prior to lung resection. Ann Thorac Surg 1995;60:603–8 [discussion: 609].
39. Olsen GN, Bolton JW, Weiman DS, Hornung CA. Stair climbing as an exercise test to predict the postoperative complications of lung resection. Two years' experience. Chest 1991;99:587–90.
40. Bolliger CT, Wyser C, Roser H, et al. Lung scanning and exercise testing for the prediction of postoperative performance in lung resection candidates at increased risk for complications. Chest 1995;108:341–8.
41. Van Nostrand D, Kjelsberg MO, Humphrey EW. Preresectional evaluation of risk from pneumonectomy. Surg Gynecol Obstet 1968;127:306–12.
42. Brunelli A, Al Refai M, Monteverde M, et al. Stair climbing test predicts cardiopulmonary complications after lung resection. Chest 2002;121:1106–10.
43. Brunelli A, Fianchini A. Stair climbing test in lung resection candidates with low predicted postoperative FEV1. Chest 2003;124:1179.
44. Brunelli A, Monteverde M, Al Refai M, Fianchini A. Stair climbing test as a predictor of cardiopulmonary complications after pulmonary lobectomy in the elderly. Ann Thorac Surg 2004;77:266–70.
45. Brunelli A, Sabbatini A, Xiume F, et al. Inability to perform maximal stair climbing test before lung resection: a propensity score analysis on early outcome. Eur J Cardiothorac Surg 2005;27:367–72.
46. Wasserman K, Whipp BJ. Exercise physiology in health and disease. Am Rev Respir Dis 1975;112:219–49.
47. Datta D, Lahiri B. Preoperative evaluation of patients undergoing lung resection surgery. Chest 2003;123:2096–103.
48. Weisman IM. Cardiopulmonary exercise testing in the preoperative assessment for lung resection surgery. Semin Thorac Cardiovasc Surg 2001;13:116–25.
49. Singh SJ, Morgan MD, Hardman AE, et al. Comparison of oxygen uptake during a conventional treadmill test and the shuttle walking test in chronic airflow limitation. Eur Respir J 1994;7:2016–20.
50. Swinburn CR, Wakefield JM, Jones PW. Performance, ventilation, and oxygen consumption in three different types of exercise test in patients with chronic obstructive lung disease. Thorax 1985;40:581–6.
51. Morgan AD. Simple exercise testing. Respir Med 1989;83:383–7.
52. Smith TP, Kinasewitz GT, Tucker WY, et al. Exercise capacity as a predictor of post-thoracotomy morbidity. Am Rev Respir Dis 1984;129:730–4.
53. Bernstein ML, Despars JA, Singh NP, et al. Reanalysis of the 12-minute walk in patients with chronic obstructive pulmonary disease. Chest 1994;105:163–7.
54. Win T, Jackson A, Sharples L, et al. Cardiopulmonary exercise tests and lung cancer surgical outcome. Chest 2005;127:1159–65.
55. Walsh GL, Morice RC, Putnam JB Jr, et al. Resection of lung cancer is justified in high-risk patients selected by exercise oxygen consumption. Ann Thorac Surg 1994;58:704–10 [discussion: 711].

56. Richter Larsen K, Svendsen UG, Milman N, et al. Exercise testing in the preoperative evaluation of patients with bronchogenic carcinoma. Eur Respir J 1997;10: 1559–65.
57. Morice RC, Peters EJ, Ryan MB, et al. Exercise testing in the evaluation of patients at high risk for complications from lung resection. Chest 1992;101:356–61.
58. Bechard D, Wetstein L. Assessment of exercise oxygen consumption as preoperative criterion for lung resection. Ann Thorac Surg 1987;44:344–9.
59. Zibrak JD, O'Donnell CR. Indications for preoperative pulmonary function testing. Clin Chest Med 1993;14:227–36.
60. Stein M, Cassara EL. Preoperative pulmonary evaluation and therapy for surgery patients. JAMA 1970;211:787–90.
61. Tisi GM. Preoperative evaluation of pulmonary function. Validity, indications, and benefits. Am Rev Respir Dis 1979;119:293–310.
62. Mitsudomi T, Mizoue T, Yoshimatsu T, et al. Postoperative complications after pneumonectomy for treatment of lung cancer: multivariate analysis. J Surg Oncol 1996;61:218–22.
63. Bolliger CT, Soler M, Stulz P, et al. Evaluation of high-risk lung resection candidates: pulmonary haemodynamics versus exercise testing. A series of five patients. Respiration 1994;61:181–6.
64. BTS guidelines: guidelines on the selection of patients with lung cancer for surgery. Thorax 2001;56:89–108.
65. Beckles MA, Spiro SG, Colice GL, Rudd RM. The physiologic evaluation of patients with lung cancer being considered for resectional surgery. Chest 2003;123:105S–14S.
66. Putnam JB Jr, Lammermeier DE, Colon R, et al. Predicted pulmonary function and survival after pneumonectomy for primary lung carcinoma. Ann Thorac Surg 1990;49:909–14 [discussion: 915].
67. Neary WD, Heather BP, Earnshaw JJ. The Physiological and Operative Severity Score for the en Umeration of Mortality and morbidity (POSSUM). Br J Surg 2003;90:157–65.
68. Copeland GP, Jones D, Walters M. POSSUM: a scoring system for surgical audit. Br J Surg 1991;78:355–60.
69. Brunelli A, Fianchini A, Gesuita R, Carle F. POSSUM scoring system as an instrument of audit in lung resection surgery. Physiological and operative severity score for the enumeration of mortality and morbidity. Ann Thorac Surg 1999;67:329–31.
70. Melendez JA, Carlon VA. Cardiopulmonary risk index does not predict complications after thoracic surgery. Chest 1998;114:69–75.
71. Ferguson MK, Durkin AE. A comparison of three scoring systems for predicting complications after major lung resection. Eur J Cardiothorac Surg 2003;23:35–42.
72. Nici L, Donner C, Wouters E, et al. American Thoracic Society/European Respiratory Society statement on pulmonary rehabilitation. Am J Respir Crit Care Med 2006;173:1390–413.
73. Troosters T, Casaburi R, Gosselink R, Decramer M. Pulmonary rehabilitation in chronic obstructive pulmonary disease. Am J Respir Crit Care Med 2005;172: 19–38.
74. Rationale and design of The National Emphysema Treatment Trial: a prospective randomized trial of lung volume reduction surgery. The National Emphysema Treatment Trial Research Group. Chest 1999;116:1750–61.
75. Bartels MN, Kim H, Whiteson JH, Alba AS. Pulmonary rehabilitation in patients undergoing lung-volume reduction surgery. Arch Phys Med Rehabil 2006;87. S84–8 [quiz: S89–90].

76. Ries AL, Make BJ, Lee SM, et al. The effects of pulmonary rehabilitation in the national emphysema treatment trial. Chest 2005;128:3799–809.
77. Moy ML, Ingenito EP, Mentzer SJ, et al. Health-related quality of life improves following pulmonary rehabilitation and lung volume reduction surgery. Chest 1999;115:383–9.
78. Sekine Y, Chiyo M, Iwata T, et al. Perioperative rehabilitation and physiotherapy for lung cancer patients with chronic obstructive pulmonary disease. Jpn J Thorac Cardiovasc Surg 2005;53:237–43.
79. Bobbio A, Chetta A, Ampollini L, et al. Preoperative pulmonary rehabilitation in patients undergoing lung resection for non-small cell lung cancer. Eur J Cardiothorac Surg 2008;33:95–8.
80. Fielding JE. Smoking: health effects and control (1). N Engl J Med 1985;313: 491–8.
81. Nakagawa M, Tanaka H, Tsukuma H, Kishi Y. Relationship between the duration of the preoperative smoke-free period and the incidence of postoperative pulmonary complications after pulmonary surgery. Chest 2001;120:705–10.
82. Vaporciyan AA, Merriman KW, Ece F, et al. Incidence of major pulmonary morbidity after pneumonectomy: association with timing of smoking cessation. Ann Thorac Surg 2002;73:420–5 [discussion: 425–6].
83. Sardari Nia P, Weyler J, Colpaert C, et al. Prognostic value of smoking status in operated non-small cell lung cancer. Lung Cancer 2005;47:351–9.
84. Gillinov AM, Heitmiller RF. Strategies to reduce pulmonary complications after transhiatal esophagectomy. Dis Esophagus 1998;11:43–7.
85. Whooley BP, Law S, Murthy SC, et al. Analysis of reduced death and complication rates after esophageal resection. Ann Surg 2001;233:338–44.
86. Nagawa H, Kobori O, Muto T. Prediction of pulmonary complications after transthoracic oesophagectomy. Br J Surg 1994;81:860–2.
87. Bailey SH, Bull DA, Harpole DH, et al. Outcomes after esophagectomy: a ten-year prospective cohort. Ann Thorac Surg 2003;75:217–22 [discussion: 222].
88. Hulscher JB, van Sandick JW, de Boer AG, et al. Extended transthoracic resection compared with limited transhiatal resection for adenocarcinoma of the esophagus. N Engl J Med 2002;347:1662–9.
89. Fan ST, Lau WY, Yip WC, et al. Prediction of postoperative pulmonary complications in oesophagogastric cancer surgery. Br J Surg 1987;74:408–10.
90. Ferguson MK, Durkin AE. Preoperative prediction of the risk of pulmonary complications after esophagectomy for cancer. J Thorac Cardiovasc Surg 2002;123: 661–9.
91. Avendano CE, Flume PA, Silvestri GA, et al. Pulmonary complications after esophagectomy. Ann Thorac Surg 2002;73:922–6.

Hemoptysis and Thoracic Fungal Infections

Seema Kapur, MD, Brian E. Louie, MD, FRCSC*

KEYWORDS

• Hemoptysis • Fungal infections • Management

At some point in their career, most general surgeons will be faced with a patient with hemoptysis or a thoracic fungal infection. These patients usually present with minor symptoms and require a stepwise comprehensive evaluation to determine appropriate treatment. A minority of patients present acutely or in extremis from either condition. Because of the rarity of these presentations, a well-organized algorithm to approach the patient is the best preparation. This article is divided into 2 separate but related sections. First, the management of hemoptysis is discussed in terms of the initial assessment, stabilization, proper use of diagnostic options, and treatment choices. Second, the spectrum of fungal diseases is reviewed, the role of surgery in fungal disease is identified, and the surgical treatments are discussed.

HEMOPTYSIS

The term hemoptysis comes from the Greek words haima meaning blood, and ptysis meaning spitting. Hemoptysis is defined as the expectoration of blood originating from the tracheobronchial tree or lung parenchyma and is seen as a manifestation of many lung diseases. For the physician it is a worrisome symptom that warrants further assessment. For the patient, it is fraught with fear and anxiety not only regarding the eventual diagnosis but also from the possibility of loss of airway and asphyxiation.

Most often, patients describe coughing up small amounts of blood and respiratory distress from contamination of the remaining lung with blood. Fortunately exsanguinating hemoptysis is extremely rare, but asphyxiation secondary to aspirated blood can occur with a significant bleed.

Definitions

Hemoptysis is usually categorized by the severity of bleeding. Most definitions focus on massive hemoptysis and assume that anything less is nonmassive or limited. Quantitatively, more than 600 mL of bleeding in 24 hours is considered massive but

---

Division of Thoracic Surgery, Swedish Cancer Institute and Medical Center, Suite 850, 1101 Madison Street, Seattle, WA 98105, USA
* Corresponding author.
E-mail address: brian.louie@swedish.org

Surg Clin N Am 90 (2010) 985–1001
doi:10.1016/j.suc.2010.06.006
0039-6109/10/$ – see front matter © 2010 Elsevier Inc. All rights reserved.

surgical.theclinics.com

quantities from 200 to 1000 mL in 24 hours have been reported in the literature.[1] However, these definitions fail to consider that the volume of the tracheobronchial tree is approximately 200 mL. Thus, a more clinical and practical definition of massive hemoptysis is any bleeding that results in a threat to life because of airway or hemodynamic compromise by bleeding.

Anatomy and Pathophysiology

The lungs receive their blood supply via the pulmonary arterial circulation and the systemic bronchial arteries. Other systemic vessels may also supply the lung in pathologic conditions secondary to neovascularization from inflammation or in rare cases from congenital anomalies. These vessels are often found coursing from the chest wall across the pleural space to the lung or in the inferior pulmonary ligament and can be the source of ongoing hemoptysis.

Although the pathogenesis of hemoptysis varies with the underlying cause, more than 90% of cases of hemoptysis result from disruption of branches of the bronchial arteries. Bronchial artery neovascularization is the most common pathway and generally results from diseases that cause pulmonary arteriole occlusion from hypoxic vasoconstriction, thrombosis, or vasculitis. In diseases like bronchitis, cystic fibrosis, or fungal infections, acute or chronic inflammation creates tortuous ectatic vessels through neovascularization that are prone to rupture. Pulmonary parenchymal necrosis from necrotizing pneumonia or infarction of lung from pulmonary embolism, inflammatory and immunologic vasculitides can also lead to hemorrhage by exposing the capillary bed.

Erosion into a major pulmonary vessel, trauma to a major vessel, or rupture of a pulmonary vessel is generally responsible for massive and frequently fatal hemoptysis. Direct erosion of mass or cavitary lesions occur in tuberculosis, fungal infections, cancer; or pulmonary arteriovenous or bronchovascular fistulas. One recently identified cause of massive hemoptysis is the use of bevacizumab, a vascular endothelial growth factor angiogenesis inhibitor, that when used in the treatment of central squamous carcinomas of the lung may result in massive hemoptysis.[2] Traumatic disruption may result from a deceleration injury, penetrating trauma, or occasionally from perforation after pulmonary artery catheterization. Spontaneous rupture of the pulmonary artery branches may complicate secondary pulmonary hypertension associated with mitral stenosis or congenital heart disease. These conditions lead to secondary pulmonary hypertension.

Epidemiology and Cause

Tuberculosis remains the most common cause of hemoptysis worldwide with an estimated 2 billion people infected and another 5% to 10% expected to develop the disease. In contrast, the most common causes of hemoptysis in the United States and other industrialized countries are bronchitis, bronchiectasis, and bronchogenic carcinoma, with prevalences of 2% to 40%. Acute and chronic bronchitis are estimated to account for up to 50% of cases. Comparatively, 20% of patients with bronchogenic carcinoma develop hemoptysis at some point and only 7% have hemoptysis as their initial presentation.[3]

Massive hemoptysis, in both developed and undeveloped countries, is most commonly caused by chronic infection from tuberculosis, mycetoma, or lung abscess. The subset of patients with exsanguinating hemoptysis (less than 1% of cases) most commonly have bronchovascular fistulization from cavitary infections or neoplasm. The underlying cause is never found in 15% to 30% of cases and is referred to as cryptogenic or idiopathic hemoptysis.[4]

A list of common causes of hemoptysis is shown in **Box 1**.

Approach to the Patient with Hemoptysis

The principles guiding the approach to hemoptysis are best conceived in terms of the acuteness or severity of the bleeding. Hence, bleeding that is intermittent, slow, and

---

Box 1
Common causes of hemoptysis

Infectious

Chronic bronchitis

Bronchiectasis

Mycobacterium

    Tuberculosis

    Atypical mycobacterial

Necrotizing pneumonia

Lung abscess

Fungus

    Invasive

    Mycetoma

Cystic fibrosis

Neoplasms

Primary lung tumors

Secondary lung tumors

Cardiovascular

Mitral stenosis

Severe left heart failure

Pulmonary embolism/infarction

Arteriovenous malformation

Bronchovascular fistula

Autoimmune

Wegener granulomatosis

Systemic lupus erythematosis

Goodpasture disease

Idiopathic pulmonary hemosiderosis

Trauma

Pulmonary contusion/laceration

Pulmonary artery catheter rupture

Miscellaneous

Foreign body

After needle biopsy

Coagulation disorders

minimally symptomatic can be approached from the perspective of identifying the source and planning for control of the lesion. Depending on whether the patient is minimally or moderately symptomatic from nonmassive hemoptysis, the evaluation may be conducted on an outpatient or inpatient basis. However, if the patient presents with massive or life-threatening hemoptysis, emergency control of the airway and bleeding along with intensive care unit resuscitation should precede any definitive attempts at treating the underlying lesion. Therefore, the management of patients with hemoptysis is a concerted and multidisciplinary effort.[5]

The management of massive hemoptysis has changed in the last 2 decades.[6,7] Earlier literature has focused on emergent surgical intervention. This resulted in significant mortality and morbidity associated with the instability of the patient at presentation. Even if they survived the operation, they often had a higher incidence of long-term ventilator dependence and pneumonia related to contamination of the contralateral lung.[5] Presently, the recommended strategy is for initial nonoperative management and stabilization followed by delayed definitive operation as necessary.[5,8] This has led to a significant decrease in the mortality associated with surgical management of severe hemoptysis.

Massive or life-threatening hemoptysis

In managing life-threatening hemoptysis, the immediate goal of the surgeon is to preserve life by protecting the healthy lung from aspiration/contamination and then control hemorrhage. More specifically, we prefer to sequentially address each goal outlined here before moving on to the next:

- Airway and lung protection
- Hemorrhage control
- Determine definitive care plan.

The initial management in life-threatening or massive hemoptysis begins with a quick assessment of the patient to determine the status of the airway, breathing, and circulation. The patient should be positioned with the presumed bleeding side down to protect the unaffected lung from further soilage with blood while preparing for more definitive management. If the location of bleeding is undetermined or the patient prefers, an upright position is also acceptable during this initial phase of management. Concurrently, a focused history and physical examination to elicit a potential list of causes is performed as well as a chest radiograph, routine laboratory tests, coagulation profile, arterial blood gas analysis, and cross match. We insist on 2 large-bore intravenous lines, supplemental oxygen, and a Foley catheter. Broad-spectrum antibiotic therapy should be initiated, as there is usually an acute bacterial infectious component to most cases of severe hemoptysis whatever the underlying primary pathology.

Airway and lung protection Airway and lung protection is established in the operating room for obvious reasons. The room is set up so that both rigid and flexible endoscopy can be performed simultaneously; 2 suction setups, ice-cold saline, and jet ventilation should also be available.

In ongoing exsanguinating hemoptysis, rigid bronchoscopy allows gross removal of clots and debris. Room temperature saline injection can help break up clots. Alternating suction and irrigation should permit the lateralization of the source of bleeding to be right or left. The rigid scope is then advanced into the nonbleeding side, the airways are toileted, and ventilation and oxygenation resumed via the ventilating bronchoscope.

In cases of severe hemoptysis that seems to have stopped, a flexible, therapeutic bronchoscope can be used through a large-bore endotracheal tube (ETT, >8.0 Fr). This allows careful assessment of the situation, determine laterality, and hopefully provide some evidence of the cause. In such a situation, we strongly suggest not to proceed at the bedside in the intensive care unit but recommend going to the operating room with rigid endoscopy equipment in the room if needed.

If bronchoscopy is not immediately available, a single-lumen endotracheal intubation is preferred to protect the airway and, particularly if the bleeding is coming from the right, can be used to isolate the healthy lung from the presumed bleeding side while preparations are made. At this stage of management, a double-lumen ETT has limited usefulness because it requires more skill for accurate placement, is too small to adequately suction blood and clots, and has a tendency to dislodge.[9]

Methods of hemorrhage control There are a variety of methods described to control hemorrhage in the airway. The choice of control depends on the situation, the cause, and the local expertise available. Once the airway is controlled and the healthy lung protected, the next step is to control of the hemorrhage. The airway remains a shared domain with anesthesia and clear concise communication is essential. Our initial attempt at hemorrhage control is with ice-cold saline lavage. The iced saline is instilled in 50- to 100-mL aliquots followed by suctioning and repeated until there is noticeable improvement. At regular intervals, the nonbleeding airway is reintubated with the rigid scope to allow oxygenation. A mixture of 1 mL of 1:1000 epinephrine diluted in 10 mL of normal saline can be used in conjunction with the iced saline.

The next step in management depends on the success of these initial efforts and if there is a clearer understanding of the cause. When hemostasis cannot be achieved, there are concerns for rebleeding and because there is a need to prevent further soilage of the contralateral lung, it is preferable to isolate both lungs. Placement of an endobronchial blocker on the bleeding side in this setting offers several advantages. First, blockers can be advanced under visualization to the bleeding site for effective tamponade. Second, they are easy to use and can be left in place. Third, when used with a standard ETT, flexible bronchoscopy and toilet of the opened airways can still be performed. The blocker (a size 4–8 Fr Fogarty balloon catheter depending on the size of the airway to be occluded) is guided into the airway alongside the ETT. Under bronchoscopic guidance, it is directed into the culprit segmental or lobar bronchus and inflated with saline to control further airway flooding. If bleeding has stopped and we have significant concerns about rebleeding, we leave the deflated balloon in the appropriate main stem to be rapidly inflated if rebleeding ensues.

There are commercial endobronchial catheter kits that come with a 3-way port that attaches to the ETT and allows the ventilator, blocker, and bronchoscope to enter via independent ports. Because the blocker is placed within the ETT, it needs to be secured to the ETT to prevent dislodgement and it limits the ability to pass a bronchoscope. Also minor displacements of the patients' neck may dislodge the blocker so it is important to keep the patient's head and neck immobile.

The alternatives to using a bronchial blocker for lung separation are to use an extra long ETT and selectively intubate the main stem bronchus of the unaffected side or place a double-lumen ETT. Selective main stem intubation is a helpful technique to control an emergency situation particularly for right-sided hemorrhages, but when the situation is controlled we prefer the bronchial blocker option. A double-lumen tube has limited usefulness in our experience as discussed earlier, but in select situations it may be helpful.

If the bleeding has been localized and controlled, we leave the patient intubated and move toward more definitive control of the bleeding and treatment because recurrent bleeding is common even after adequate initial control. For most patients, the next step is to undergo bronchial artery embolization (BAE). Its use was first reported by Remy and colleagues[10] in 1973 and subsequent reports[11–13] have documented its safety and efficacy in controlling massive hemoptysis, either as a definitive therapy in nonsurgical candidates or as a temporizing and stabilizing technique before definitive resection.

Thorough knowledge of the often variable bronchial artery anatomy is required of the angiographer; a single left and right bronchial artery is present only one-third of the time. Once the optimal approach vessel is cannulated, findings consistent with hemoptysis such as extravasation, hypertrophic and tortuous arteries, aneurismal change, neo- and hypervascularity, and shunting into the pulmonary artery or vein are identified.[14] In our experience, prior endoscopic identification of the side or better, the lobar site of bleeding, helps the angiographer in the search for the culprit feeding vessel(s).

Embolization can be performed with absorbable gelatin sponge or polyvinyl alcohol particles between 325 and 500 μm. Initial control is effective with a 70% to 98% cessation of bleeding. However, long-term control is suboptimal with a 10% to 50% recurrence within 4 years. Rebleeding may be caused by recanalization of the embolized vessel, progression of disease, or continued neovascularization. Results can be improved with repeat embolization although most authorities agree that the role of BAE is palliative and temporary with a need for subsequent control of the underlying disease with antibiotics or surgery. BAE is usually safe. The most serious morbidity is spinal cord ischemia, which has been reported to occur up to 6.5% in earlier series.[11]

Persistent bleeding after BAE warrants additional angiographic evaluation. Communication with the angiographer is important at this stage because the site of bleeding may be arising from nearby bronchial vessels because of neovascularization, aberrant systemic arteries arising from the intercostal or internal mammary arteries; or through vascular adhesions resulting from the chronic inflammatory pulmonary process. Rarely, a pulmonary arterial study may be required to identify the source of bleeding.[15,16]

Improvements in imaging technology and comfort with computed tomography (CT) angiography as a diagnostic tool are likely to continue changing the management of hemoptysis. CT angiography not only has the ability to diagnose pulmonary parenchymal lesions but can also identify possible candidates for upfront pulmonary arterial superselective vasoocclusion.[17] Findings on CT angiography that indicate pulmonary arterial involvement includes the presence of pseudoaneurysm, aneurysmal change of the pulmonary vessels, and the presence of a pulmonary artery close to or in the lesion.

Although BAE has become the mainstay of treatment, there are several endobronchial treatments that can be used particularly if here is an endoluminal cause for the bleeding. Topical thrombin or thrombin fibrinogen instilled via small bore catheter inserted into the suction port is reportedly effective.[18] Topical coagulation with laser photocoagulation (Nd:YAG and less commonly CO_2) have been used with success rates of more than 60% or the argon plasma coagulator via the bronchoscope can also be used. Endobronchial brachytherapy in high doses (10–12 Gy/h for a total of 500–4000 Gy) has also been used for control of hemoptysis with a more than 85% success rate. Endobronchial cryotherapy is a useful technique that not only causes tissue destruction (for endoluminal masses) but also has the additional benefit of vasoconstriction and microthrombosis.[9]

Definitive management Definitive management of the patient with hemoptysis depends on the patient's performance status, the underlying cause, and likelihood for recurrence.

Nonsurgical management For patients who are medically inoperable or when the disease causing the hemoptysis is nonsurgical, treating the underlying disease is crucial. For patients with malignant disease, radiation therapy offers the possibility of treating both the cancer and the neovascularization. The underlying premise is to obliterate the microvascular blood supply resulting from neovascularization and reduce the likelihood of recurrent hemoptysis.[19] Similarly, radiation has been used to treat hemoptysis resulting from aspergilloma.[20] Intracavitary administration of amphotericin B for aspergilloma has also been shown to successfully arrest hemorrhage and potentially dissolve the mycetoma with minimal complications.[21] However, the cavity remains in most patients.[21]

Surgical management Most often, the techniques described earlier succeed in controlling the bleeding. This gives the surgeon time to further evaluate the patient's risk for surgery and allow optimization of the patient's condition for surgery. If initial attempts to control bleeding and stabilize the patient are unsuccessful, emergency surgery is an option. However, the decision to take the patient to the operating room emergently must be made with knowledge of at least the laterality and optimally the lobar location of the lesion. Once considered the most effective method for controlling hemoptysis, surgery has been approached more recently with caution and knowledge that there are improved outcomes with initial nonsurgical management and patient optimization.

If surgical resection for hemoptysis is contemplated, the patient must be medically operable in terms of physiology and meet the indications for resection of the specific disease. The most common indications for surgical resection are mycetoma, cancer, bronchiectasis, and tuberculosis.[6] If cancer is the underlying reason, the patient must be resectable for cure because radiation therapy offers hemorrhage control.

Summary
The management of hemoptysis has entered a new era in which endoscopic and angiographic treatments have become the mainstay of initial therapy. Conversion of an emergent situation to a semi-elective surgical problem by first using these methods for controlling the bleeding has significantly reduced the operative mortality and morbidity of surgery done for hemoptysis.

FUNGAL DISEASE IN THE THORACIC CAVITY

Similar to hemoptysis, significant and symptomatic fungal disease in the thoracic cavity that requires surgical involvement is uncommon. However, with the incidence of fungal infections of the lung and/or superinfection of the lung with fungal elements continuing to increase, there is a need for surgeons to understand, diagnose, and treat fungal diseases in the thoracic cavity. In this section, the pathophysiology is discussed, the fungal pathogens and their thoracic manifestations are reviewed, and the role of surgery in various situations involving fungal diseases is discussed.

Pathophysiology
Fungal organisms are ubiquitous in the environment and entry into the human host via normal respiration is probably more frequent and undetected than we assume. Usually the response by otherwise immune competent patients with normal lungs is

asymptomatic or at most a mild flulike illness with spontaneous clearance and return to usual function.

Two predominant groups of patients are at risk of developing pulmonary fungal disease: those with impaired immunity, congenital or acquired, and those with chronically diseased or destroyed lungs. The former group of patients includes transplant recipients on immune suppressive therapy, patients who have cancers on receiving chemotherapy, and patients with immune deficiency syndromes who are more susceptible to otherwise innocuous or opportunistic pathogens. Neutropenia or prolonged corticosteroid use for any reason are also clear risk factors for development of fungal infections, as are chronic illnesses such as diabetes and severely debilitated patients in the intensive care unit with long-term intubation or long courses of broad-spectrum antibiotic coverage.[8,22] Patients with structurally abnormal lungs or chronic lung conditions have impaired local bronchopulmonary defense mechanisms and as such are at a higher risk for the development of a fungal infection.

Presentation and Pathogens

The presentation of thoracic and pulmonary mycoses can be varied and confusing. The spectrum of disease produced by these organisms ranges from patients who are asymptomatic with only radiographic findings of enlarged hilar and mediastinal nodes or calcified lymph nodes or granulomas from prior fungal infection to life-threatening hemoptysis.[23] In between, patients present with nonspecific minor pulmonary symptoms such as cough, pleurisy, dyspnea, and hemoptysis that may be associated with self-limited flulike symptoms. The more common endemic fungal infections in North America and their presentation and surgical treatment are shown in **Table 1**.

Evaluation and Investigations

Evaluation of the patient suspected of having a thoracic pulmonary fungal infection begins with a thorough history and physical examination focusing on onset and spectrum of symptoms, contacts, exposures, travel, recent medications, and comorbidities. Special attention is paid to the patient's recent travel history and migratory patterns. There are several regions in North America known to have a high prevalence of a particular type of fungal exposure in the population. The Mississippi River, Ohio and Missouri valleys are renowned for histoplasmosis; the southeastern United States and Kenora, Ontario, Canada for blastomycosis; and the southwestern desert areas of Nevada and Arizona along with the San Joaquin Valley in California for coccidiomycosis.

Physical examination is often unremarkable. Chest examination may reveal lymphadenopathy. Extrapulmonary manifestations of fungal disease should also be assessed; for instance for a patient being evaluated for *Cryptococcus*, it would be important to do a thorough neurologic examination to rule out a brain abscess. Laboratory studies include complete blood count, blood and sputum cultures for bacteria, fungus, and acid-fast bacilli. Cultures are best obtained via induced sputum that is immediately sent to the laboratory. Serial sputum studies can be done to increase the yield and they should be kept in culture for 4 to 8 weeks. Serologic testing is available for individual species. These are either fungal antigens or antibody response tests. Serial serologies done at least 3 weeks apart are sometimes more helpful in gauging the effect of treatment or disease progression. More recently, molecular diagnosis via polymerase chain reaction is becoming available although it requires specialized equipment and personnel.[24]

Although many patients undergo plain chest radiographs, a diagnostic CT scan of the chest is the most useful. The radiological findings of respiratory fungal infections mimic other lung diseases and has limited value in predicting the causative organism. These signs include interstitial infiltrates, bronchopneumonia, consolidation, segmental pneumonia, solitary or multiple nodules, masses, cavitary lesions, and pleural effusion. Cavitary lesions may be observed on chest radiograph although a CT scan can reveal crescentic cavitation much earlier than a chest radiograph. This radiologic sign is classic for an aspergilloma although intracavitary fungus balls caused by other filamentous fungi may present in a similar manner.[25]

In the immune-compromised population, proving the diagnosis of a fungal infection is difficult because of the lack of positive cultures and reduced sensitivity of serologic tests in patients receiving prophylactic or empiric antifungal agents.[23,26] CT scans may be highly suggestive, but with the myriad of potential diagnoses in these patients a biopsy will likely be necessary to confirm a fungal infection.[27] Endoscopic biopsy or needle biopsy is preferred as the initial attempt at diagnosis before moving on to surgical biopsy given the limited reserve and frailty of some of these patients.

When the clinical, radiological, and microbiological data do not help to differentiate between infection and colonization, fiberoptic bronchoscopy with bronchoalveolar lavage and transbronchial biopsies or CT-guided percutaneous transthoracic lung biopsies are undoubtedly the most reliable methods for establishing a certain diagnosis and for defining the species of fungi responsible for infection in suspected respiratory fungal infections. These methods are not problematic to perform in immunocompetent individuals. However, their use in patients with poor general health and a tendency to bleed, such as hematologic patients and recipients of bone marrow transplantation must be placed in the context of other diagnostic options. Transthoracic biopsies have the added downside of a 5% to 15% incidence of subsequent pneumothorax with chest drain placement.[27]

The Role of Surgery in Thoracic Fungal Infections

The role for surgery in thoracic fungal infections ranges from diagnostic biopsies to surgical resection of the infected area, usually a lobe. Because of the rarity of the disease as well as the overlap in signs and symptoms, the surgeon must carry a heightened awareness that fungus may play a role in the presentation of the patient.

Diagnostic biopsy

Within the thoracic cavity, patients may present for biopsy in 1 of 3 different instances: lymphadenopathy, parenchymal lung changes, and mediastinal fibrosis.

Lymphadenopathy Patients presenting with persistent mediastinal and/or hilar lymphadenopathy (**Fig. 1**) often have a complex medical history that does not allow a more narrow differential diagnosis. Biopsy is usually requested to rule out metastatic cancer or other diseases such as sarcoidosis, lymphoma, and tuberculosis. Fungal infections are not obviously suspected upfront, but may become a priority when caseating granulomas are identified. Appropriate intraoperative cultures of nodal biopsies should include not only mycobacterial diseases but also fungal cultures and stains.

The usual access in this situation is by cervical mediastinoscopy. Occasionally, with palpable adenopathy, supraclavicular or scalene node biopsies may be diagnostic. Although Wang needle transbronchial biopsies or endobronchial ultrasound techniques have been described for these situations, we have found that these techniques are limited to aspiration cytology and require significant cytologic experience to confidently assign a fungal diagnosis while determining that the long list of differential causative agents are not present.

Table 1
Summary of common fungal pathogens and disease processes

	Histoplasmosis	Coccidiomycosis	Blastomycosis	Cryptococcosis	Aspergillosis	Candidiasis	Actinomycosis
Common Organism	*Histoplasma capsulatum*	*Coccidioides immitis*	*Blastomyces dermatitidis*	*Cryptococcus neoformans*	*Aspergillus fumigatus*	*Candida albicans*	*Actinomyces israelii*
Geography	Ohio, Missouri, Mississippi valleys; caves in southeast United States and Mexico	Southwestern United States and Mexico	Mississippi and Ohio river valley and southeast US	Ubiquitous	Ubiquitous	Ubiquitous	Ubiquitous
Acute presentation	Flulike illness Diffuse lymphadenopathy with hepatosplenomegaly	Valley fever: pneumonitis, erythema nodosum and arthalgias, ARDS	Flulike illness		Dyspnea, fever unresponsive to antibiotics, hemoptysis and pulmonary infiltrates	Tracheobronchitis Pneumonia/ pulmonary abscess	Chest pain, sputum, cough
Chronic presentation		Pneumonia Meningitis Arthritis	Cutaneous, genitourinary tract, meningeal, skeletal symptoms		Allergic bronchitis Aspergilloma		Skin fistulae with sulfur granules, pleural effusions, empyema
Imaging acute	Consolidations SPN Diffuse nodules	LL consolidation Pleural effusions Subpleural nodules	LL consolidations Noncavitating solitary mass	LL consolidation	LL consolidation Halo sign	Diffuse infiltrates or masses	LL nodular density, mediastinal lymphadenopathy

Imaging chronic	Upper lobe cavities in chronic active disease; Hilar and mediastinal lymphadenopathy with calcified granulomata	Calcified granulomata; Upper lobe thin-walled cavitation; Loculated effusions	Upper lobe fibronodular opacities; Thin-walled cavitation	Air crescent sign			Cavitating lesions; may also involve pleura, chest wall or spine
Special features	Fibrosing mediastinitis; Broncholithiasis; Pericarditis	Disseminated disease in Filipino, African American men, immunocompromised or pregnant patients	Lesions rarely calcify	Tropism for vessel walls; 50% patients with aspergilloma get hemoptysis	10% develop meningitis after removal of lung lesion	Cause in 72% of fungal infections	Reclassified as a bacterium
Treatment	Amphotericin B; Itraconazole	Amphotericin B	Amphotericin B; Ketoconazole	Ketoconazole	Amphotericin B; Ketoconazole	Fluconazole; Caspofungin	High-dose penicillin
Hemoptysis	Rare	Sometimes	Rare	Common	Sometimes	Common	Sometimes
Reason for surgical intervention	SPN, r/o malignancy	SPN, r/o malignancy; Cavitary disease, rupture, hemoptysis	Diagnosis	Diagnosis		Drainage of pulmonary abscess	Diagnosis, drainage of abscess, empyema

Abbreviations: ARDS, acute respiratory distress syndrome; LL, lower lobar; r/o, rule out; SPN, solitary pulmonary nodule.

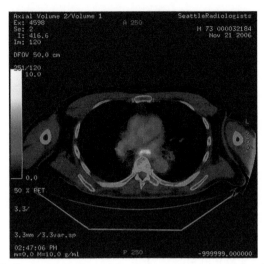

Fig. 1. Hypermetabolic mediastinal and hilar adenopathy demonstrated on positron emission tomography scan. Mediastinoscopy biopsies demonstrated caseating granulomas and fungal organisms consistent with coccidiomycosis.

Parenchymal lung disease Parenchymal lung changes such as tree and bud appearance, interstitial fibrosis, or lobar consolidation are more amenable to bronchoscopic diagnosis. Often targeted transbronchial biopsies are diagnostic without the need to proceed to surgical biopsy. If a surgical parenchymal biopsy is required, most lesions are amenable to a video-assisted thoracoscopic (VATS) approach.[28] The advantage of VATS is that more tissue is collected for culture and analysis, it allows for thorough evaluation of the pleural space particularly if an effusion is present and it allows for assessment of the pulmonary parenchymal surface. When dealing with a diffuse parenchymal process, it is preferable to obtain 2 or 3 wedge biopsies to provide the pathologist with adequate tissue sampling especially if there is no obvious microbial agent. Staple lines from each wedge resection are sent for fungal and bacterial culture. Using the VATS approach yields a specific diagnosis 67% of the time in patients with unexplained pulmonary infiltrates with 1 in 5 diagnosis attributed to aspergillosis.[29]

Mediastinal disease More complicated scenarios such as mediastinal granuloma or fibrosing mediastinitis (**Fig. 2**) are often difficult to diagnose with core biopsies because adequate sampling is not achieved. Surgical biopsies are often requested to provide additional tissue for culture and staining. Mediastinal biopsies can be obtained either through anterior mediastinotomy on the side that is most affected or occasionally, VATS is used to obtain a biopsy at multiple sites including the anterior mediastinum. Surgical input may also be required to prevent or treat complications such as superior vena cava syndrome, fistulas to airway or esophagus, or hemoptysis from erosion into great vessels. These complications, however, are beyond the scope of this article.

Solitary pulmonary nodule
The development of a solitary pulmonary nodule may occur in the healing phase of infection primarily with histoplasmosis, coccidiomycosis (**Fig. 3**), and aspergillous. The radiographic picture is often confused with a primary bronchogenic neoplasm[30] because there is often associated mediastinal adenopathy and a remote smoking

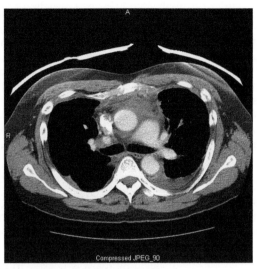

Fig. 2. Mediastinal fibrosis secondary to histoplasmosis.

history. Because most patients are asymptomatic, the only clue pointing toward a fungal cause may be a remote history of a nonspecific flulike illness or recent travel to an endemic area.

The solitary pulmonary nodule is best approached assuming that the patient has a bronchogenic carcinoma. A search for prior chest radiographs or CT scans to compare with current imaging occasionally demonstrates a stable nodule on serial imaging and prevents unnecessary biopsies. More commonly, the patient undergoes a thorough evaluation including positron emission tomography scan and pulmonary

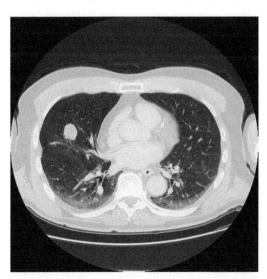

Fig. 3. Solitary pulmonary nodule in a heavy smoker. Wedge resection demonstrated a coccidioma.

function testing in preparation for surgery. Traditional teaching in the management of solitary pulmonary nodules recommended against presurgical biopsies. However, with improvements in interventional radiology, core needle biopsy and the introduction of endobronchial ultrasound and navigational bronchoscopy biopsy, fewer and fewer patients are taken to the operating room without a biopsy.[30] Biopsy proven fungal nodules require antifungal treatment and surveillance until resolution of the nodule. When the biopsies are nondiagnostic or the patient prefers excision, these lesions are general amenable to VATS wedge resection and in rare instances lobectomy provides a definitive diagnosis and treatment. Fully resected nodules do not require systemic fungal treatment unless there is evidence of invasive fungal infection on final pathology.

Hemoptysis

Patients who present with hemoptysis and are suspected of having a pulmonary fungal infection are initially treated as outlined in the first section of this article. Surgery may be considered for persistent or recurrent hemoptysis.

Mycetoma

Mycetoma or cavitary fungal disease is of 2 types. The first is related to primary infection by fungal inoculum and starts as a walled cyst. This is a simple mycetoma and has less devastating consequences. The fraction of living versus dead fungus determines the growth rate and stable cavitary disease can be observed safely. The second is a complex mycetoma (**Fig. 4**), which arises in a preexisting cavitary lesion from a myriad of diseases. Most common is tuberculosis, however other causes include sarcoidosis, bullous emphysema, and fibrosis. These may become stable or may grow causing hemoptysis, pneumonia, or disseminated infections.

Surgical resection of a mycetoma is usually a challenging procedure even for the most experienced thoracic surgeon. The mere presence of a mycetoma in general is an indication to consider resection. Lesions that are symptomatic, enlarging, or potentially concerning for eventual complications of ongoing erosion and growth should be considered for resection in suitable patients. The goals of surgery include the removal of all fungal elements including the damaged lung parenchyma while preserving the normal functioning lung. When surgical resection is undertaken in selected patients and in a controlled manner, the results are generally excellent.[6,26,31–36]

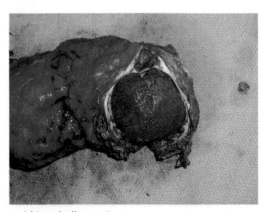

Fig. 4. Aspergilloma within a bullae cavity.

The most challenging are the patients who are immunocompromised. However, recent studies have shown the feasibility of early and aggressive operative management in this population. Early surgical intervention for removal of persistent cavitation has been shown to reduce/eliminate active disease and relapse of fungal infection, especially after bone marrow transplant. In addition, secondary prophylaxis is dependent on accurate diagnosis, which sometimes is only possible via histopathologic evaluation of infected tissue. Also, early removal of mycetoma or residual cavitary disease eliminates the high mortality (50%) of first-time hemoptysis in this subset of patients. Although the surgical mortality and major complication rate for surgical intervention are both 10%, it is acceptable in this high-risk population.[26,29,37–40]

Invasive pulmonary fungal disease

Invasive fungal infection is usually associated with an immunocompromised state and can complicate stem cell transplant in up to 9% of cases.[41] Medical management with antifungals has been the primary mode of treatment yet the results have been disappointing. The role of surgery remains highly controversial. The indications to consider surgical resection in patients with invasive fungal infection include disease adjacent to a single large vessel or pericardium, a single lesion as the source of hemoptysis, erosion into the pleural space or ribs, and localized extrapulmonary lesions.[29]

Transplant patients who develop an invasive pulmonary fungal infection generally present early after their primary procedure with symptoms of systemic illness and minor hemoptysis. Radiographically, there is rapid progression of a nodular pulmonary infiltrate that begins to coalesce into a mass with a hazy margin (halo sign) or a cavitary mass with a crescent-shaped area of hyperlucency (air crescent sign) within a parenchymal opacity.

Surgical resection can be considered in these individuals with characteristic radiologic findings who are confined to a lobe or anatomic unit. Early resection with perioperative intravenous antifungal therapy has been recommended because a reasonable surgical mortality can be achieved with 1-year survival of 65%.[36,38] The comparative 1-year survival with medical therapy remains disappointing at 5% or less.[38]

SUMMARY

Thoracic fungal infections represent a broad spectrum of disease from simple radiographic findings to life-threatening mycetomas with massive hemoptysis. Most fungal infections are mild and self-limited. The minority of infections that are symptomatic are likely to involve the surgeon in terms of diagnostic biopsy, surgical resection, and lifesaving procedures.

REFERENCES

1. Patterson AG, Cooper JD, Deslauriers J, et al, editors, Pearson's thoracic and esophageal surgery, vol. 1. 3rd edition. Philadelphia: Churchill-Livingstone; 2008.
2. Sandler AB, Schiller JH, Gray R, et al. Retrospective evaluation of the clinical and radiographic risk factors associated with severe pulmonary hemorrhage in first-line advanced, unresectable non-small-cell lung cancer treated with Carboplatin and Paclitaxel plus bevacizumab. J Clin Oncol 2009;27(9):1405–12.
3. Hirshberg B, Biran I, Glazer M, et al. Hemoptysis: etiology, evaluation, and outcome in a tertiary referral hospital. Chest 1997;112(2):440–4.
4. Corder R. Hemoptysis. Emerg Med Clin North Am 2003;21(2):421–35.

5. Shigemura N, Wan IY, Yu SC, et al. Multidisciplinary management of life-threatening massive hemoptysis: a 10-year experience. Ann Thorac Surg 2009; 87(3):849–53.

6. Andrejak C, Parrot A, Bazelly B, et al. Surgical lung resection for severe hemoptysis. Ann Thorac Surg 2009;88(5):1556–65.

7. Jougon J, Ballester M, Delcambre F, et al. Massive hemoptysis: what place for medical and surgical treatment. Eur J Cardiothorac Surg 2002;22(3):345–51.

8. Silveira F, Paterson DL. Pulmonary fungal infections. Curr Opin Pulm Med 2005; 11(3):242–6.

9. Karmy-Jones R, Cuschieri J, Vallieres E. Role of bronchoscopy in massive hemoptysis. Chest Surg Clin N Am 2001;11(4):873–906.

10. Remy J, Voisin C, Ribet M, et al. [Treatment, by embolization, of severe or repeated hemoptysis associated with systemic hypervascularization]. Nouv Presse Med 1973;2(31):2060 [in French].

11. Uflacker R, Kaemmerer A, Neves C, et al. Management of massive hemoptysis by bronchial artery embolization. Radiology 1983;146(3):627–34.

12. Rabkin JE, Astafjev VI, Gothman LN, et al. Transcatheter embolization in the management of pulmonary hemorrhage. Radiology 1987;163(2):361–5.

13. Kato A, Kudo S, Matsumoto K, et al. Bronchial artery embolization for hemoptysis due to benign diseases: immediate and long-term results. Cardiovasc Intervent Radiol 2000;23(5):351–7.

14. Yoon W, Kim JK, Kim YH, et al. Bronchial and nonbronchial systemic artery embolization for life-threatening hemoptysis: a comprehensive review. Radiographics 2002;22(6):1395–409.

15. Remy-Jardin M, Wattinne L, Remy J. Transcatheter occlusion of pulmonary arterial circulation and collateral supply: failures, incidents, and complications. Radiology 1991;180(3):699–705.

16. Khalil A, Parrot A, Nedelcu C, et al. Severe hemoptysis of pulmonary arterial origin: signs and role of multidetector row CT angiography. Chest 2008;133(1): 212–9.

17. Remy-Jardin M, Bouaziz N, Dumont P, et al. Bronchial and nonbronchial systemic arteries at multi-detector row CT angiography: comparison with conventional angiography. Radiology 2004;233(3):741–9.

18. Tsukamoto T, Sasaki H, Nakamura H. Treatment of hemoptysis patients by thrombin and fibrinogen-thrombin infusion therapy using a fiberoptic bronchoscope. Chest 1989;96(3):473–6.

19. Hatlevoll R, Karlsen KO, Skovlund E. Endobronchial radiotherapy for malignant bronchial obstruction or recurrence. Acta Oncol 1999;38(8):999–1004.

20. Falkson C, Sur R, Pacella J. External beam radiotherapy: a treatment option for massive haemoptysis caused by mycetoma. Clin Oncol (R Coll Radiol) 2002; 14(3):233–5.

21. Giron J, Poey C, Fajadet P, et al. CT-guided percutaneous treatment of inoperable pulmonary aspergillomas: a study of 40 cases. Eur J Radiol 1998;28(3):235–42.

22. Lass-Florl C, Salzer GM, Schmid T, et al. Pulmonary Aspergillus colonization in humans and its impact on management of critically ill patients. Br J Haematol 1999;104(4):745–7.

23. Chen KY, Ko SC, Hsueh PR, et al. Pulmonary fungal infection: emphasis on microbiological spectra, patient outcome, and prognostic factors. Chest 2001;120(1): 177–84.

24. Buchheidt D, Hummel M. Aspergillus polymerase chain reaction (PCR) diagnosis. Med Mycol 2005;43(Suppl 1):S139–45.

25. Chong S, Lee KS, Yi CA, et al. Pulmonary fungal infection: imaging findings in immunocompetent and immunocompromised patients. Eur J Radiol 2006;59(3): 371–83.

26. Ali R, Ozkalemkas F, Ozcelik T, et al. Invasive pulmonary aspergillosis: role of early diagnosis and surgical treatment in patients with acute leukemia. Ann Clin Microbiol Antimicrob 2006;5:17.

27. Kim K, Lee MH, Kim J, et al. Importance of open lung biopsy in the diagnosis of invasive pulmonary aspergillosis in patients with hematologic malignancies. Am J Hematol 2002;71(2):75–9.

28. Gossot D, Validire P, Vaillancourt R, et al. Full thoracoscopic approach for surgical management of invasive pulmonary aspergillosis. Ann Thorac Surg 2002;73(1):240–4.

29. Theodore S, Liava'a M, Antippa P, et al. Surgical management of invasive pulmonary fungal infection in hematology patients. Ann Thorac Surg 2009;87(5):1532–8.

30. Meyerson SL, Wilson J, Smyth S. Tissue diagnosis of new lung nodules in patients with a known malignancy. Am J Surg 2009;198(6):841–5.

31. Al-Kattan K, Ashour M, Hajjar W, et al. Surgery for pulmonary aspergilloma in post-tuberculous vs. immuno-compromised patients. Eur J Cardiothorac Surg 2001;20(4):728–33.

32. Babatasi G, Massetti M, Chapelier A, et al. Surgical treatment of pulmonary aspergilloma: current outcome. J Thorac Cardiovasc Surg 2000;119(5):906–12.

33. Erdogan A, Yegin A, Gurses G, et al. Surgical management of tuberculosis-related hemoptysis. Ann Thorac Surg 2005;79(1):299–302.

34. Kim YT, Kang MC, Sung SW, et al. Good long-term outcomes after surgical treatment of simple and complex pulmonary aspergilloma. Ann Thorac Surg 2005; 79(1):294–8.

35. Mabeza GF, Macfarlane J. Pulmonary actinomycosis. Eur Respir J 2003;21(3): 545–51.

36. Matt P, Bernet F, Habicht J, et al. Predicting outcome after lung resection for invasive pulmonary aspergillosis in patients with neutropenia. Chest 2004;126(6): 1783–8.

37. Sole A, Salavert M. Fungal infections after lung transplantation. Curr Opin Pulm Med 2009;15(3):243–53.

38. Robinson LA, Reed EC, Galbraith TA, et al. Pulmonary resection for invasive Aspergillus infections in immunocompromised patients. J Thorac Cardiovasc Surg 1995;109(6):1182–96 [discussion: 1196–7].

39. Nosari A, Ravini M, Cairoli R, et al. Surgical resection of persistent pulmonary fungus nodules and secondary prophylaxis are effective in preventing fungal relapse in patients receiving chemotherapy or bone marrow transplantation for leukemia. Bone Marrow Transplant 2007;39(10):631–5.

40. Habicht JM, Passweg J, Kuhne T, et al. Successful local excision and long-term survival for invasive pulmonary aspergillosis during neutropenia after bone marrow transplantation. J Thorac Cardiovasc Surg 2000;119(6):1286–7.

41. Thursky K, Byrnes G, Grigg A, et al. Risk factors for post-engraftment invasive aspergillosis in allogeneic stem cell transplantation. Bone Marrow Transplant 2004;34(2):115–21.

The Solitary Pulmonary Nodule: Approach for a General Surgeon

Nicholas R. Thiessen, MD[a], Ross Bremner, MD, PhD[b],*

KEYWORDS

- Solitary pulmonary nodule • Lung cancer • Investigation
- Surgery • CT scan

Out, damn'd spot! out, I say!—Lady Macbeth: Macbeth Act 5, scene 1.

A pulmonary nodule is a radiographic spheroidal opacity in the lung, defined by the Fleishner Society as being less than 3 cm in diameter.[1] Opacities greater than 3 cm are most commonly malignant and are referred to as a "mass," although this cutoff is somewhat arbitrary, and in practice lesions above 3 cm are often referred to as nodules. Most nodules are incidental radiographic findings, but because the finding may represent an asymptomatic malignancy, the primary goal is to exclude carcinoma. The lung is a common site for metastatic lesions, and primary lung cancer is one of the most common cancers in the western world and accounts for the highest mortality of all cancers.[2] Yet the lung is the site of far more benign radiographic abnormalities than malignant. **Table 1** provides a list of the more common causes of a solitary pulmonary nodule (SPN). In this era of frequent computed tomographic CT scanning the "incidental nodule" is now an epidemic radiologic finding, and how to determine the benign versus malignant nature of the lesion is becoming increasingly important. It is estimated that more than 60 million CT scans were performed in the United States in 2006, a 3-fold increase from a decade earlier, and this is on the rise.[3] Most frequently, the General Surgeon encounters a patient with a solitary nodule when a chest radiograph or CT scan is done for other reasons such as routine preoperative testing or the workup for trauma. This article provides a logical approach to the workup and management of an SPN in this setting.

This work was supported by a grant from St Joseph's Foundation.

[a] Department of surgery, Joseph's Hospital and Medical Center, 350 West Thomas Road, Phoenix, AZ 85013, USA

[b] Center for Thoracic Disease, The Heart and Lung Institute, St Joseph's Hospital and Medical Center, 500 West Thomas Road, Suite 500, Phoenix, AZ 85013, USA

* Corresponding author.

E-mail address: Ross.bremner@chw.edu

Surg Clin N Am 90 (2010) 1003–1018

doi:10.1016/j.suc.2010.07.002

0039-6109/10/$ – see front matter © 2010 Elsevier Inc. All rights reserved.

surgical.theclinics.com

Table 1
Possible cause of the solitary pulmonary nodule (SPN)

Malignant Lesions	Benign Lesions	Infectious	Noninfectious	Congenital	Other
Bronchogenic carcinoma	Hamartoma	Tuberculosis	Rheumatoid arthritis	Bronchogenic cyst	Hematoma
Small cell carcinoma	Lipoma	Atypical mycobacterial infection	Wegener granulomatosis		Bronchiolitis obliterans organizing pneumonia
					Pseudotumor
Large cell carcinoma	Fibroma	Histoplasmosis	Sarcoidosis		
Adenocarcinoma		Coccidioidomycosis			Pulmonary infarction
Squamous carcinoma		Blastomycosis			Amyloidoma
Solitary metastasis		Aspergilloma			Rounded atelectasis
Carcinoid		Ascaris			Mucoid impaction
Other/rare		Dirofilariasis			
		Echinococcal cyst			
		Bacterial abscess			

THE SUBCENTIMETER NODULE

Because of the sensitivity and high resolution of CT scanning, small nodules less than 1 cm are not uncommon. These nodules represent a unique subgroup, and it is appropriate to deal with these at the outset of this article because most of the ensuing discussion reflects the approach to nodules 1 to 3 cm in size. Subcentimeter nodules are less likely to be malignant and are often difficult to diagnose, mostly because lesions of this size are below the resolution of positron emission tomography (PET) and because it is difficult to biopsy these lesions with fine-needle aspiration (FNA). These small nodules should be watched with serial scanning unless there is some other factor that increases the potential for malignancy, such as the history of the patient or the CT characteristics of the nodule. Highly suspicious peripheral nodules can undergo FNA biopsy, navigation brochoscopy biopsy, or video-assisted thoracoscopic surgery (VATS), but occasionally special techniques are required to find these nodules at surgery, such as preoperative dye or needle localization techniques. From initial screening trials, it is clear that the risk of malignancy for lesions greater than 5 mm in size is very low (probably <1%) and that repeat scanning in 12 months is probably adequate. For lesions 6 to 9 mm in size, the risk for malignancy is in the range of 5% to 10%, and repeat scanning in 3 to 6 months is justified[4] with a longer period before the next scan if the nodule remains unchanged (**Fig. 1**). The limitations of all of these diagnostic tests are described below.

RADIOGRAPHIC FEATURES

Although a nodule may be found on a chest radiograph, it is a more common finding on CT scan because a CT scan is much more sensitive in detecting small abnormalities. Further, the initial response to a radiograph abnormality (and radiologist recommendation on radiograph report) is to perform a CT scan. Characteristics of a CT scan can help us with the prediction of a benign or malignant diagnosis. Lesions with rounded smooth margins are more likely to be benign. Examples include granulomatous inflammation or a hamartoma (**Fig. 2**). A spiculated margin or one with a corona radiata sign (very fine linear strands extending 4–5 mm outward from the nodule) is more commonly associated with a malignant lesion (**Fig. 3**). A scalloped border is associated with an intermediate probability of cancer, whereas a smooth border is more suggestive of a benign diagnosis.[5]

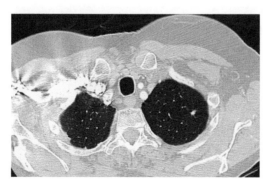

Fig. 1. A 56-year-old man with a 6-mm nodule stable over 1 year. Awaiting repeat scan at 2 years. This nodule would be difficult to biopsy by either FNA or VATS and is below the limits of resolution for PET.

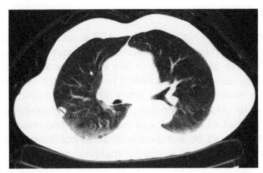

Fig. 2. Rounded nodule discovered incidentally at CT-angiogram performed for chest pain in a 52-year-old. Lesion found to be a hamartoma.

Calcification within a nodule suggests a benign lesion (**Fig. 4**A, B), although some malignant nodules may contain a calcific pattern. Patterns of calcification are more easily observed on CT scans than on plain-film radiographs.[6] With CT considered the reference standard, plain-film radiographs of the chest have a sensitivity, specificity, and positive predictive value of 50%, 87%, and 93%, respectively, for identifying calcification, thus stressing the value of CT scanning in better characterizing these lesions. A laminated or central pattern is typical of a granuloma, whereas a classic "popcorn" pattern is most often seen in hamartomas (**Fig. 5**). In approximately half the cases of hamartoma, high-resolution CT scan can show a definitive pattern of fat and cartilage. Calcification patterns that are stippled or eccentric have been associated with cancer.[5]

Cavitary lesions with a thick wall are most frequently associated with a malignancy, whereas thin-walled cavities usually denote an infectious cause, but this is not always the case (**Fig. 6**).[7] A fungus ball or mycetoma is usually seen as a density in a cavity, but this does not exclude the possibility of carcinoma. Pulmonary emboli most frequently produce wedge-shaped lesions that abut the pleura, but chronic infarcts can mimic cancer.

CT scan with dynamic enhancement is used in many centers and has been proven to be highly sensitive but not specific for the diagnosis of malignancy. Absence of lung

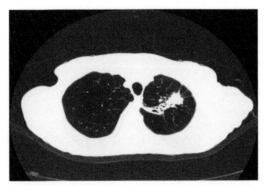

Fig. 3. Left upper lobe speculated nodule in a 70-year-old smoker with emphysema. Needle biopsy showed poorly differentiated adenocarcinoma. This lesion is associated with a more central fibrotic scar.

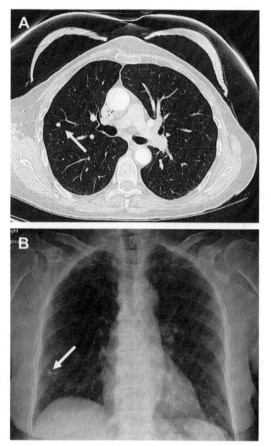

Fig. 4. (*A, B*) An incidental solitary pulmonary nodule (*arrow*) in a 50-year-old woman. Soft-tissue windows showed this to be a calcified nodule, and a remote chest radiograph showed it to be present 5 years previously. No follow-up is required. This illustrates the value of obtaining old radiographs.

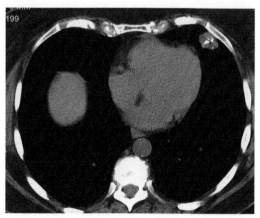

Fig. 5. Soft tissue window CT scan showing popcorn calcification in a hamartoma.

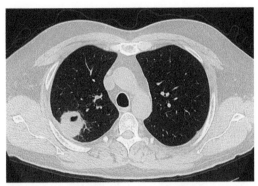

Fig. 6. A thick-walled cavity that showed spherules typical of coccidioidomycosis on needle biopsy, which resolved with antifungal treatment. Thick-walled cavitary lesions may also represent a malignancy with a necrotic center.

nodule enhancement on dynamic CT scan, however, is strongly predictive of benignity. CT scan with contrast can help diagnose vascular lesions, especially of arteriovenous malformations (**Fig. 7**).

OLD RADIOGRAPHS

Apart from examining the radiographic characteristics of the lesion, the first step in evaluating an SPN is to try to find old radiographs with which to compare the presence and size of the lesion. A little effort exerted to locate an old chest radiograph or CT scan may save a lot of time, money, and possibly further interventional studies, because nodules that stable over time are usually benign (see **Fig. 4**). The size of malignant lesions usually change over time although the same can be seen with infectious or inflammatory lesions. The Schwartz formula looks at the doubling time based on initial measurements and compares that to subsequent measurements to help predict the doubling time of the lesion (**Fig. 8**).

The doubling time has been studied for different primary lung tumors and differs based on cell type. On average, the doubling time for adenocarcinomas is 163.3 days, squamous cell carcinoma 80.3 days, small cell carcinoma 69.2 days, and large

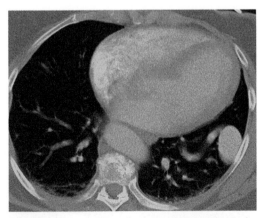

Fig. 7. Arteriovenous malformation with prominent associated vessel seen best with intravenous contrast.

$$DT = \frac{t \log 2}{\log V_t / V_o} = \frac{t \log 2}{\log \dfrac{a_t \times b_t{}^2}{a_o \times b_o{}^2}}$$

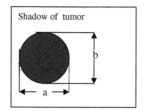

Fig. 8. The Schwartz formula can be used to assess the doubling time of the mass to help understand the risk of malignancy in a nodule that changes over time. This formula is not used in most centers, although newer CT software that evaluates volumetric change over time will likely be helpful in the future. (*Adapted from* Usuda K, Saito Y, Sagawa M, et al. Tumor doubling time and prognostic assessment of patients with primary lung cancer. Cancer 1994 Oct 15;74(8):2239–44; with permission.)

cell carcinomas 66.8 days.[8] Some studies have shown that the doubling time for squamous cell carcinoma can be faster than that for adenocarcinoma.[8–12] However, there is a wide range of variation of doubling times for malignant nodules in the literature, ranging from 20 to 300 days.[4,13–15] The current recommendation is that a pulmonary nodule that is unchanged on serial radiographic imaging over 2 years is most likely benign and does not need further workup. There are 2 major caveats with this recommendation: (1) some lesions such as carcinoid tumors, atypical adenomatous hyperplasia, and bronchioloalveolar carcinoma (adenocarcinoma in situ [AIS]) may remain relatively stable for periods longer than 2 years but do have a more sinister prognosis than benign lesions if and when change occurs; and (2) solitary lung nodules are often missed by even experienced chest radiologists and may not be reported in either a previous or a current study. "Missed" lesions are not uncommon. In a recent retrospective study[4,16] of 40 patients with non–small cell lung cancers that were initially missed on chest radiograph, the median diameter of the lesions was 1.9 cm, and 85% of the lesions were peripheral in location. In the Mayo Lung Project,[17] 45 of 50 screening-detected peripheral carcinomas were visible on previous radiographs when reviewed in retrospect. One attempt to improve on this with automated computer-assisted recognition of nodules., This system is yet to be perfected but currently has the ability to enhance a primary radiologist interpretation.[18]

ASSESSMENT OF THE PROBABILITY OF MALIGNANCY

In this article, details of the benefits of the various diagnostic tests are discussed, but it is essential that at the outset some idea of the probability of malignancy be assessed. A 15-year-old patient with a smooth, rounded 1-cm nodule clearly has a different probability of having a malignancy than that of a 70-year-old patient with a strong smoking history with a 2.5-cm spiculated nodule. In an effort to predict probability of malignancy, various models have been put forth and some formulas developed, including the use of artificial intelligence and neural networks. The Mayo Clinic used a database of 419 patients and regression analysis to develop an equation to estimate the risk of malignancy. This complex algorithm is available for use,[19–21] but it has been found to provide little benefit over prediction by expert clinicians.[22] It is thus important to have radiologic abnormalities reviewed by experts who deal with lung cancer on a daily basis or by a committee of experts such as is found in a multidisciplinary tumor board. A basic starting point can be obtained by using the characteristics given in **Table 2**.[5]

Table 2
Characteristics to help assess likelihood of malignancy in the SPN

Variable	Risk of Cancer		
	Low	Intermediate	High
Diameter of nodule (cm)	<1.0	1–2	>2
Age (y)	<45	45–60	>60
Smoking status	Never smoked	Current smoker (<20 cigarettes/day)	Current smoker (>20 cigarettes/day)
Smoking-cessation status	Quit >7 y ago or never smoked	Quite <7 y ago	Never quit
Characteristics of nodule margins	Smooth	Scalloped	Corona radiata or spiculated

Definite benign calcification and nodules unchanged for more than 2 years are excluded from this probability table.

Because most lung cancers are found in patients with a significant smoking history, this is naturally an important consideration when predicting risk of cancer. The risk for developing lung cancer decreases with time after smoking cessation but never equals that of the nonsmoker, denoting a lifetime increased risk. There has been an increase in the incidence of lung cancer in patients with no smoking exposure, and in some patients, this increasing incidence may be related to significant second-hand smoke exposure. Further, radon and asbestos exposure are not easily known or quantified and represent other significant risk factors for lung cancer.

A noncalcified indeterminate nodule on chest radiograph should prompt a CT scan for reasons mentioned earlier. By using the CT appearance, the history of the patient, and any available previous imaging studies, a reasonable conclusion can be reached regarding the need for further studies. Watchful waiting versus a further intervention is the next decision to be made and is usually made on the basis of malignant potential. Further intervention may include a trial of antibiotics or antifungals, PET scanning, bronchoscopy with possible biopsy or brushings, navigation bronchoscopy, CT-guided transthoracic biopsy, or thoracoscopic biopsy or wedge resection (VATS).

A useful algorithm to approach the suspicious SPN is shown in **Fig. 9** and is useful when used in conjunction with **Table 2**. This is only a guideline, and ideally advice on how to proceed should come from a multidisciplinary group as described earlier. The authors think that any suspicious nodules should at least be reviewed by a thoracic surgeon who understands the complexities of further testing and surgical intervention and who sees these nodules on a daily basis.

Watchful Waiting

Watchful waiting of a solitary pulmonary nodule is a reasonable option in patients with a low risk for malignancy and/or in those who are at high risk for complications of surgical resection. Patients should understand that watchful waiting may delay the diagnosis of a malignancy, but this is of uncertain clinical significance if a repeat scan is done within 3 to 6 months. Any lesion that increases in size should undergo an attempt at tissue diagnosis, either by needle biopsy or by surgery. For stable lesions, repeat scans at 3-month intervals for the first year and then 6-month intervals

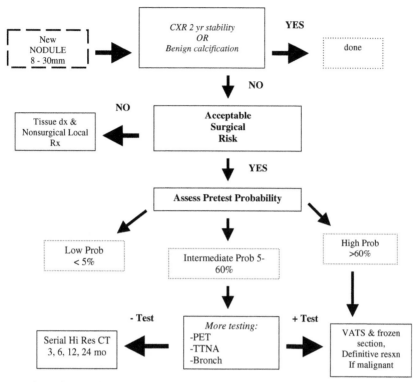

Fig. 9. Algorythm to help guide workup of the patient who is found to have an SPN. (*Adapted from* Ost D, Fein AM, Feinsilver SH. Clinical practice. The solitary pulmonary nodule. N Engl J Med 2003 Jun 19;348(25):2535–42; with permission.)

for the second year have been recommended by the American Radiological Society, but this would certainly be excessive for a very small nodule (>5 mm) and would expose the patient to a significant amount of radiation. Radiation risk from repeat CT scanning is significant, and the irradiation from a single CT of the chest without contrast is approximately equal to about 350 postero-anterior chest radiographs.[3] The risk from radiation exposure is related to the potential for development of a subsequent malignancy, a paradox in the sense that multiple CT scans performed to diagnose cancer may increase the risk of subsequent malignancy. It is estimated that approximately 2% of all cancers diagnosed in the United States today are a result of previous radiation exposure from radiologic studies.[3] This is especially important with respect to young patients who carry this radiation risk for a longer period. Because lung cancer is unusual in young patients, multiple CT scans should be avoided in patients younger than 35 years if at all possible.

The protocols for CT scanning of the chest are not uniform, and the radiation exposure is variable from center to center. Further, few institutions practice the latest techniques of limiting radiation exposure to As Low As Reasonably Achievable.[23] Variables such as current modulation, preprogramming, and real-time feedback mechanisms can be used to minimize radiation exposure.[24] When following a particular nodule with watchful waiting, another means of limiting exposure is to scan the patient only in the area of the nodule and not the entire chest. This method is an underutilized practice but should be considered when multiple scans may be necessary in the patient.

Antibiotics and Antifungals Followed by Repeat CT Scan

If a lesion is thought to be infectious in nature, a trial of empiric antimicrobial therapy is an option. The use of this therapy is not to be encouraged if a patient is asymptomatic or if the lesion does not have features strongly suggestive of an infectious process such as coccidioidomycosis. Indiscriminate use of antibiotics results in the development of more resistant organisms and may provide time for a malignancy to grow. CT features of air-containing lesions, satellite nodules, air bronchograms and thin-walled cavitation are often indicative of an infectious process, but these features can also be misleading. Cocci titres may be useful in a patient with systemic symptoms from an endemic area, but these titres are often negative, and a dormant cocci granuloma may not stimulate a significant antibody response. The malignant lesion most likely to emulate an infectious process is bronchiolo-alveolar carcinoma, which is a noninvasive cancer that can spread thoughout the lungs by lepidic growth (along alveolar septae). This lesion will most likely be referred to in the future as AIS for reasons beyond the scope of this article. Apart from development of resistant organisms, long-term antibiotics have known side effects, as does long-term azole treatment for fungal infections (antitestosterone effect and liver toxicity). **Fig. 10** shows a patient with an air-containing lesion treated for 4 months with various antimicrobials before having a needle biopsy after significant progression of the lesion. Biopsy revealed an adenocarcinoma in a background of bronchioloalveolar carcinoma. This lesion required a bilobectomy with a portion of the upper lobe to be removed. A lesser resection may have been possible if a biopsy was performed earlier. As a corollary, though, any patient with an inflammatory lesion that progresses or does not regress after antimicrobial therapy should undergo further evaluation.

PET Scanning

Scanning the patient with fluorodeoxyglucose (^{18}F-FDG) enables some understanding of the metabolism of the lesion; however, many inflammatory lesions can also give positive results and lesions such as sarcoid, active tuberculosis, histoplasmosis,

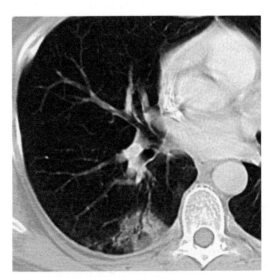

Fig. 10. An air-containing lesion typical of an inflammatory process or a bronchiolar-alveolar carcinoma (adenocarcinoma in situ).

rheumatoid nodules, and coccidioidomycosis can mimic cancer with high-standard uptake values. The high specificity of PET-CT allows one to consider an SPN with low uptake of ^{18}F-FDG to be benign if the lesion is at least 1 cm in size. False negative results have been reported in the literature, mostly with primary pulmonary malignancies, such as carcinoids, bronchioloalveolar carcinomas, adenocarcinomas with a predominantly bronchioloalveolar carcinoma component, and malignant SPNs of less than 10 mm in diameter.[25–28] PET has been found to have a sensitivity and specificity of approximately 87% and 83%, respectively, for assessing an SPN,[29] but knowledge of the reasons behind false positive and false negative results is important when using PET as a diagnostic tool. The great value of PET in lung cancer is in staging rather than diagnosis because PET provides information regarding mediastinal nodal involvement and distant metastatic disease. However, PET is commonly used to add diagnostic information and is often suggested on a CT report by the radiologist, prompting the automatic request for a PET. These reports are expensive studies that may be unhelpful and, worse, can be misleading. Again bronchioloalveolar carcinoma (or AIS) may not have much avidity for PET, resulting in a false sense of security with a negative scan. Similarly, a carcinoid tumor may have little FDG avidity and may subsequently be overlooked.[26,28] Nonetheless, it is an additive test that can be used to help assess metabolic activity, and as such cold lesions offer the opportunity to watch the lesion because it is more likely to be benign. FDG-PET may be most cost effective when the probability assessment is low, but the CT scan findings of a lesion are suspicious. Of importance though, a negative PET scan result does not completely exclude a diagnosis of malignancy, and further follow-up is required.

Bronchoscopy

Bronchoscopy can be diagnostic for more centrally located malignant lesions, typically squamous or small cell cancers. (**Fig. 11**). The most common lung cancers are peripheral adenocarcinomas or metastatic lesions, and for these lesions, standard bronchoscopy with washings or transbronchial biopsy is less likely to provide a diagnosis. In an attempt to improve on the diagnostic yield for more peripheral lesions, navigational bronchoscopy has recently been developed.[30] This technology uses electromagnetic fields and sophisticated software to allow directional positioning of

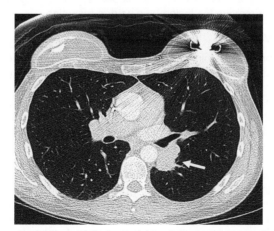

Fig. 11. A 2.8-cm central hilar nodule (*arrow*) in a 44-year-old woman with recently diagnosed breast cancer. Transbronchial biopsy showed this lesion to be a separate non–small cell lung adenocarcinoma ultimately removed by surgery.

the end of the bronchoscope (akin to a global positioning system for the lung) so that a biopsy needle can be inserted directly into the peripheral area of interest for biopsy. Although this technology is innovative and has the potential to be added to our armamentarium of diagnostic tests, it is not yet widely available, is expensive, and is not appropriately reimbursed for the time and effort involved and requires the aid of significant intravenous sedation or general anesthesia. It does offer the potential benefit of a biopsy of a peripheral lesion with a reduced chance of pneumothorax compared with a CT-guided transthoracic biopsy. Feducial gold seeds can also be placed at the time of navigational bronchoscopy if the lesion proves to be malignant and stereotactic radiation is planned.

CT-Guided Needle Biopsy

This biopsy is one of the most commonly used and beneficial means for evaluating peripheral nodules. Either FNA or core-needle biopsies can be obtained, with the former having less risk of pneumothorax and the latter having a higher diagnostic yield. The risk of pneumothorax is in the range of 25%, but only a small percentage of these require further intervention such as chest tube or pigtail drainage. The risk of pneumothorax increases with deeper lesions, lesions near fissures, and in patients with lung disease, such as fibrosis or emphysema. Some of these patients with a postneedle biopsy pneumothorax may require hospitalization, and if there is significant underlying emphysema, a prolonged air leak may ensue. Needle biopsy provides a definitive diagnosis if the specimen contains malignant cells, typical infectious particles such as coccidioidomycosis spherules, or fat and cartilage as seen in a hamartoma, but often the diagnosis is indeterminate or inconclusive. Care must be taken in interpreting these results, and these results should not be interpreted as the lesion being benign. Once the suspicion for malignancy has reached the point of prompting an invasive needle biopsy, the investigator should not stop until a definitive diagnosis has been obtained. The diagnostic accuracy of transthoracic needle biopsy varies depending on size. Small lesions (<15 mm) have a diagnostic accuracy of approximately 74%, whereas larger lesions (>15 mm) have a greater potential for accurate diagnosis (96%).[25] The accuracy of transthoracic needle aspiration for definitive diagnosis of benign disease is reported to be 50%[25] to 70%.[31] An inconclusive needle biopsy should prompt either another attempt at needle biopsy or surgical intervention to biopsy the lesion or remove the lesion by a wedge resection.

Thoracoscopy or VATS

Thoracoscopy represents a minimally invasive surgical means to both diagnose and potentially treat pulmonary nodules. **Fig. 9** shows which patients may be better served by early referral for surgical intervention, without submitting the patient to unnecessary further testing. The typical patient taken for a VATS wedge resection is older but healthy enough for surgery and has a strong smoking history and a radiographically suspicious peripheral lung nodule. Similarly, patients with a lung nodule who are at high risk for risk a pulmonary metastases from a locally advanced tumor of another organ system are good candidates for a diagnostic thoracoscopic wedge resection (**Fig. 12**). If the frozen section shows a nonsmall cell lung cancer, these patients can go on to have a lobectomy under the same anesthetic if this shows a non–small cell lung cancer. Patients with metastases to the lungs are usually adequately treated with wedge resections with adequate surgical margins. Surgery does have a defined associated morbidity and mortality, especially in patients with marginal pulmonary function or with other comorbidities. Simple wedge resection for diagnosis is associated with a low morbidity and usually requires only an overnight stay in the hospital, but lobectomy for cancer is

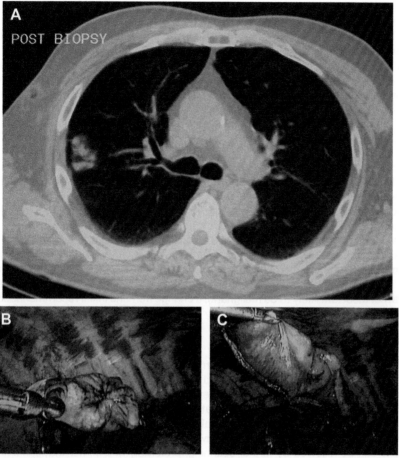

Fig. 12. (*A, B, C*) A 59-year-old man with a strong smoking history and a history of rectal carcinoma with a solitary pulmonary nodule. Needle biopsy was inconclusive (*A*). Thoracoscopy was indicated and a wedge resection was performed. Final pathology was consistent with metastatic colorectal carcinoma. In this circumstance, VATS was both diagnostic and therapeutic and required only an overnight hospital stay for the patient.

associated with a 1% to 3% chance of mortality. As with needle biopsy, severely emphysematous lungs are associated with an increased risk of complications with VATS wedge resection, particularly a prolonged air leak. Nonetheless, when applied prudently, VATS performed by experienced thoracic surgeons and thoracic anesthesiologists has a relatively low risk for complications, usually is diagnositic, and can be therapeutic in the form of a wide wedge resection or lobectomy.

SCREENING FOR LUNG CANCER BY CT SCANNING

Much of the authors' understanding of the incidence and natural history of SPNs has been gleaned from screening trials that have been performed to help diagnosis of lung cancer at an earlier stage. In theory, primary lung cancer is a tumor that may benefit greatly from screening: Lung cancer is usually asymptomatic; it is common; there is a defined high-risk group; the survival for treated early cancers far exceeds that of late-stage cancers; and screening with CT offers high resolution with a high sensitivity. Chest radiographs were found in earlier studies to be too insensitive to detect cancers at an early enough stage to improve survival, but more recent CT scanning trials have shown promise.[2] Multiple trials have been completed or are undergoing accrual, and details of these trials are beyond the scope of this article.[32,33] The trials have shown that it is able to detect more early lung cancers, most of which can be cured (usually by surgery alone), but whether we are impacting on the disease overall is still controversial. Lead-time bias and overdiagnosis are 2 epidemiologic problems that are encountered with screening.[34] The 2 greatest issues confronting us with screening are the high incidence of benign nodules found on scanning and the risks associated with either further investigation or from surgery for these nodules. The radiation exposure from numerous CT scans has been discussed, but the morbidity of investigating and treating nodules that are ultimately found to be benign is a major drawback to the screening process.

Nonetheless, these trials have provided us with better information about the natural history of small nodules, and they are providing a framework with which to better diagnose nodules at initial presentation and to define the most prudent follow-up procedures for nodules that are initially thought to have a low risk for malignancy. A good example is the new recommendation from the Early Lung Cancer Action Project group that nodules less than 5 mm in size only need a follow-up scan in 12 months (because so few of these are likely to be malignant), a change from the initial recommendation of a 3- to 6-month interval.

SUMMARY

The incidental finding of a nodular abnormality on a chest radiograph should prompt a CT scan and an attempt at locating old films. Old nodules unchanged over 2 years can usually be ignored especially if they are calcified. The patient's history, age, smoking exposure, and radiographic features of new nodules allow us to categorize the finding as to having a high, intermediate, or low risk for malignancy. High and intermediate lesions should prompt further investigation and/or surgery, whereas low-risk lesions can be followed by further scanning, preferably at a center that can limit the radiation exposure for this process. The recommendations for intervals of scanning and techniques for scanning are evolving as is the understanding of the benefit of lung cancer screening by CT scanning.

REFERENCES

1. Hansell DM, Bankier AA, MacMahon H, et al. Fleischner Society: glossary of terms for thoracic imaging. Radiology 2008;246(3):697–722.
2. Swensen SJ, Jett JR, Hartman TE, et al. Lung cancer screening with CT: Mayo Clinic experience. Radiology 2003;226(3):756–61.
3. Brenner DJ, Hall EJ. Computed tomography – an increasing source of rRadiation exposure. N Engl J Med 2007;357(22):2277–84.
4. Gould MK, Fletcher J, Iannettoni MD, et al. Evaluation of patients with pulmonary nodules: when is it lung cancer? ACCP evidence-based clinical practice guidelines (2nd edition). Chest 2007;132(Suppl 3):108S–30S.
5. Ost D, Fein AM, Feinsilver SH. Clinical practice. The solitary pulmonary nodule. N Engl J Med 2003;348(25):2535–42.
6. Berger WG, Erly WK, Krupinski EA, et al. The solitary pulmonary nodule on chest radiography: can we really tell if the nodule is calcified? AJR Am J Roentgenol 2001;176(1):201–4.

7. Iwata T, Nishiyama N, Nagano K, et al. Squamous cell carcinoma presenting as a solitary growing cyst in lung: a diagnostic pitfall in daily clinical practice. Ann Thorac Cardiovasc Surg 2009;15(3):174–7.

8. Usuda K, Saito Y, Sagawa M, et al. Tumor doubling time and prognostic assessment of patients with primary lung cancer. Cancer 1994;74(8):2239–44.

9. Geddes DM. The natural history of lung cancer: a review based on rates of tumor growth. Br J Dis Chest 1979;73:l–17.

10. Filderman AE, Shaw C, Matthay RA. Lung cancer: part I. Etiology, pathology, natural history, manifestations, and diagnostic techniques. Invest Radiol 1986; 21(1):21230–90.

11. Bone RC, Balk R. Staging of bronchogenic carcinoma. Chest 1982;82:821473–80.

12. Weiss W. Peripheral measurable bronchogenic carcinoma. Am Rev Respir Dis 1971;103:198–208.

13. Nathan MH, Collins VP, Adams RA. Differentiation of benign and malignant pulmonary nodules by growth rate. Radiology 1962;79:221–32.

14. Weiss W. Tumor doubling time and survival of men with bronchogenic carcinoma. Chest 1974;65:3–8.

15. Friberg S, Mattson S. On the growth rates of human malignant tumors: implications for medical decision making. J Surg Oncol 1997;65:284–97.

16. Shah PK, Austin JH, White CS, et al. Missed non-small cell lung cancer: radiographic findings of potentially resectable lesions evident only in retrospect. Radiology 2003;226:235–41.

17. Muhm J, Miller W, Fontana R, et al. Lung cancer detected during a screening program using four month chest radiographs. Radiology 1983;148:609–15.

18. Katsuragawa S, Doi K. Computer-aided diagnosis in chest radiography. Comput Med Imaging Graph 2007;31(4–5):212–23.

19. Swensen SJ, Silverstein MD, Ilstrup DM, et al. The probability of malignancy in solitary pulmonary nodules: application to small radiologically indeterminate nodules. Arch Intern Med 1997;157:849–55.

20. Gurney JW. Determining the likelihood of malignancy in solitary pulmonary nodules with Bayesian analysis: part I; theory. Radiology 1993;186:405–13.

21. Herder GJ, van Tinteren H, Golding RP, et al. Clinical prediction model to characterize pulmonary nodules: validation and added value of 18-F-fluorodeoxyglucose positron emission tomography. Chest 2005;128:2490–6.

22. Swensen SJ, Silverstein MD, Edell ES, et al. Solitary pulmonary nodules: clinical prediction model versus physicians. Mayo Clin Proc 1999;74:319–29.

23. McCollough CH, Primak AN, Braun N, et al. Strategies for reducing radiation dose in CT. Radiol Clin North Am 2009;47(1):27–40.

24. McCollough CH, Bruesewitz MR, Kofler JM Jr. CT dose reduction and dose management tools: overview of available options. Radiographics 2006;26(2):503–12.

25. Jeong YJ, Yi CA, Lee KS. Solitary pulmonary nodules: detection, characterization, and guidance for further diagnostic workup and treatment [review]. AJR Am J Roentgenol 2007;188(1):57–68.

26. Lowe VJ, Fletcher JW, Gobar L, et al. Prospective investigation of positron emission tomography in lung nodules. J Clin Oncol 1998;16:1075–84.

27. Erasmus JJ, McAdams HP, Patz EF Jr, et al. Evaluation of primary pulmonary carcinoid tumors using FDG PET. AJR Am J Roentgenol 1998;170:1369–73.

28. Higashi K, Ueda Y, Seki H, et al. Fluorine-18-FDG PET imaging is negative in bronchioloalveolar lung carcinoma. J Nucl Med 1998;39:1016–20.

29. Wahidi MM, Govert JA, Goudar RK, et al. Evidence for the treatment of patients with pulmonary nodules: when is it lung cancer? ACCP evidence-based clinical practice guidelines (2nd edition). Chest 2007;132(Suppl 3):94S–107S.

30. Schwarz Y, Greif J, Becker HD, et al. Real-time electromagnetic navigation bronchoscopy to peripheral lung lesions using overlaid CT images: the first human study. Chest 2006;129:988–94.

31. Klein JS, Braff S. Imaging evaluation of the solitary pulmonary nodule. Clin Chest Med 2008;29(1):15–38.

32. Henschke, CI. International early lung cancer action program: enrollment and screening protocol. New York, NY. Feb 25, 2010.

33. International Early Lung Cancer Action Program Investigators, Henschke CI, Yankelevitz DF, et al. Survival of patients with stage I lung cancer detected on CT screening. N Engl J Med 2006;355(17):1763–71.

34. Welch HG, Woloshin S, Schwartz LM, et al. Overstating the evidence for lung cancer screening: the International Early Lung Cancer Action Program (I-ELCAP) study. Arch Intern Med 2007;167(21):2289–95.

Tumors of the Mediastinum and Chest Wall

Jae Y. Kim, MD, Wayne L. Hofstetter, MD*

KEYWORDS

• Mediastinum • Mediastinal • Thymoma • Chest wall • Tumor

Tumors of the mediastinum and chest wall encompass a wide variety of histologies and may be primary, metastatic, or secondary to direct invasion from an adjacent cancer. Given the complex anatomy of the chest and proximity to vital structures, these lesions can be challenging to diagnose and treat. This review focuses on primary tumors.

MEDIASTINAL TUMORS
Mediastinal Anatomy

The mediastinum is bounded superiorly by the thoracic inlet and inferiorly by the diaphragm. For clinical purposes, the mediastinum has traditionally been divided into the anterior (or anterosuperior), middle, and posterior compartments (**Fig. 1**). There are no fascial planes between these divisions and they are in continuity with each other. Thus tumors can exist in more than 1 compartment. Nonetheless, these divisions are helpful in forming a differential diagnosis for a mediastinal mass (**Table 1**).

The anterior mediastinum lies between the sternum and the pericardium. It contains the thymus, lymph nodes, and loose connective tissue. The middle mediastinum contains the heart, the proximal great vessels, phrenic nerves, trachea, and main bronchi. The posterior mediastinum lies posterior to the pericardium and anterior to the thoracic vertebrae. It contains the esophagus, descending thoracic aorta, azygous vein, thoracic duct, and autonomic ganglia.[1] Although the heart, trachea, and esophagus lie within the mediastinum, tumors of these structures are outside the scope of this review.

ANTERIOR MEDIASTINUM

The anterior mediastinum is the most common site of primary mediastinal tumors. Anterior mediastinal masses are malignant in 59% of cases, compared with 29% for middle and 16% for posterior masses.[2] The most common primary masses in

Department of Thoracic and Cardiovascular Surgery, The University of Texas MD Anderson, 1515 Holcombe Boulevard, PO Box 0445, Houston, TX 77030, USA
* Corresponding author.
E-mail address: whofstetter@mdanderson.org

Surg Clin N Am 90 (2010) 1019–1040
doi:10.1016/j.suc.2010.06.005
0039-6109/10/$ – see front matter © 2010 Elsevier Inc. All rights reserved.

surgical.theclinics.com

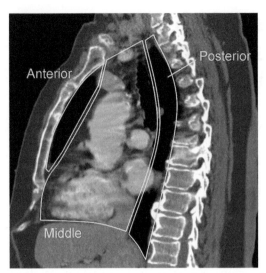

Fig. 1. A sagittal image from a computed tomography (CT) scan of the chest illustrating the anterior, medial, and posterior compartments of the mediastinum.

the anterior mediastinum are lymphomas, thymic neoplasms, germ cell tumors (GCTs), thyroid tissue, parathyroid adenomas, and cysts. Their presentations may range from an incidental finding on a radiograph to debilitating superior vena cava syndrome. Symptomatic patients are more likely to harbor malignancy. In a study of 400 patients with a primary mediastinal mass, 57% of symptomatic patients had a malignant lesion compared with only 17% of asymptomatic patients.[2] The most common symptoms were chest pain (30%), dyspnea (16%), fever/chills (20%), and cough (16%). Tumors in the anterior mediastinum are more likely to cause superior vena cava syndrome and phrenic nerve palsy.[3] The Pemberton sign is the development of facial plethora induced by raising both arms above the head. Although originally described for substernal goiter, the sign may be elicited when any mass obstructs venous outflow of the head and neck.[4]

Diagnostic Approach

A posterior-anterior (PA) and lateral chest radiograph is the initial diagnostic test that should be obtained for suspicion of any mediastinal mass. Whenever possible, the film

Table 1 Differential diagnosis for mediastinal masses	
Anterior mediastinum	Thymic neoplasm Germ cell tumor Lymphoma Thyroid Parathyroid
Middle mediastinum	Lymphoma Granuloma Cyst: bronchogenic, esophageal, pericardial
Posterior mediastinum	Neurogenic Neurenteric cyst Esophageal

should be compared with previous chest films. A computed tomography (CT) scan of the chest should be next. The CT scan provides invaluable information regarding the morphology of the mass, its extent, and relation to surrounding structures. Magnetic resonance imaging (MRI) is helpful for evaluating cystic lesions.[5] Sestamibi should be used to help localize ectopic parathyroid tissue.[6] Positron emission tomography (PET) scans are also being used more frequently for the evaluation and staging of many mediastinal tumors, including thymic neoplasms.[7]

Alpha fetoprotein (AFP) and beta human chorionic gonadotropin (beta-hCG) levels should be checked in any male with an anterior mediastinal mass. Serum calcium level should also be considered if parathyroid adenoma is suspected.

For a solid mass, the surgeon is faced with the decision of whether to obtain a biopsy or proceed with resection. A small, well-encapsulated anterior mediastinal mass on CT scan may be resected without preoperative biopsy.[8] If the mass is large or if there is the suggestion of invasion of adjacent structures, biopsy is preferred so that appropriate neoadjuvant therapy may be given.[9] In addition, if there is lymphadenopathy or if the patient presents with B symptoms, the mass should be biopsied given a suspicion of lymphoma. Fine-needle aspiration (FNA) biopsy has an accuracy of 82% for the diagnosis of mediastinal masses.[10] FNA, however, does not reliably distinguish between thymoma and lymphoma, and does not usually provide enough tissue for flow cytometry. Core needle biopsy has greater diagnostic sensitivity and specificity for mediastinal tumors. In a series of 42 patients with anterior mediastinal masses, ultrasound-guided core needle biopsy provided adequate tissue for diagnosis in 100% of the cases.[11]

In the unusual case that adequate tissue cannot be obtained from needle biopsy, then mediastinoscopy, incisional biopsy, or thoracoscopic biopsy may be performed. Parasternal mediastinotomy offers good access for incisional biopsy of most anterior masses, but must be done carefully to avoid entering the pleural cavity and disseminating the tumor with drop metastases or chest wall implants.[8] Video-assisted thoracoscopy (VATS) may also be used for biopsy but also has a risk of pleural dissemination of tumor. In general, incisional biopsy of mediastinal masses should be avoided if possible, but if necessary should be performed by surgeons who are experienced in these procedures.

Thymic Neoplasms

Thymomas are the most common anterior mediastinal tumor in adults, comprising 20% of anterior mediastinal tumors.[1,12] They have a peak incidence in the fifth and sixth decades of life.[13] Thymomas have a wide range of presentations. Many are found incidentally on imaging done for another reason. When symptoms are present cough, substernal chest pain, and dyspnea are the most common. More advanced tumors may present with findings consistent with superior vena cava syndrome, phrenic nerve paralysis, pleural effusion, or airway obstruction.[14,15] Many paraneoplastic syndromes are also associated with thymomas, most commonly myasthenia gravis and red cell aplasia.[14,16] Paraneoplastic syndromes should be screened for in any patient with suspected thymoma because they have important anesthetic and perioperative implications. Myasthenia gravis occurs in 30% to 65% of patients with thymoma. Conversely, 75% of patients with myasthenia gravis have some thymic abnormality, but only 15% have thymomas.[16] Most patients with thymomatous myasthenia gravis (70%–100%) have improvement in their neurologic symptoms after thymectomy and between 30% and 70% may attain complete remission.[17,18]

The most commonly used staging system for thymoma is the modified Masaoka staging system, which has been shown to correlate well with survival (**Table 2**).[19,20]

Table 2
Five-year survival rates for Masaoka stage

Stage		5-Year Survival (%)
I	Completely encapsulated; no microscopic capsular invasion	93–100
II	Microscopic invasion into capsule or macroscopic invasion into surrounding fatty tissue or mediastinal pleura	86–95
III	Macroscopic invasion into adjacent organs	56–70
IV	Pleural or pericardial dissemination (IVa) Lymphatic or hematogenous spread (IVb)	11–50

Data from Masaoka A, Monden Y, Nakahara K, et al. Follow-up study of thymomas with special reference to their clinical stages. Cancer 1981;48:2485; Schneider PM, Fellbaum C, Fink U, et al. Prognostic importance of histomorphologic subclassification for epithelial thymic tumors. Ann Surg Oncol 1997;4:46.

The World Health Organization (WHO) classification system for thymic neoplasms is less commonly used, but has also been shown to correlate with survival.[21,22] Invasive thymomas are often described as malignant thymomas, but they should not be confused with thymic carcinomas, which are a distinct histologic entity with more aggressive behavior.[23] Thymic carcinoids are included in the WHO classification with thymic carcinomas, but are biologically more similar to poorly differentiated neuroendocrine tumors. Like thymic carcinomas, they are aggressive tumors with potentially poor overall prognosis.[24] The mainstay of therapy is complete resection when possible.

On CT scan, the typical appearance of a thymoma is an encapsulated mass with smooth contours (**Figs. 2** and **3**). Thymic carcinomas are more heterogeneous with irregular borders and often show evidence of invasion into adjacent structures.[23] In addition, thymic carcinomas are more fluorodeoxyglucose-avid on PET.[7]

Complete surgical resection is the goal and leads to the best prognosis for patients with thymic tumors.[13] Median sternotomy, either partial or complete, has been the traditional approach, and provides excellent exposure to the tumor as well as potentially involved great vessels. Thoracoscopic resection has also been used, primarily for early stage tumors and myasthenia gravis.[25] A transcervical approach may also be used for early stage tumors less than 4 cm in size.[8] Regardless of the approach, the most important principle is removal of the entire tumor and thymus without spillage.

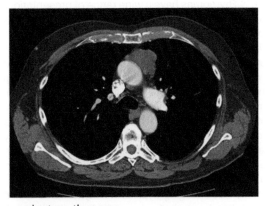

Fig. 2. CT scan of an early stage thymoma.

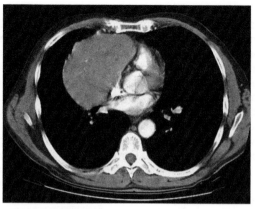

Fig. 3. CT scan of an invasive thymoma.

For Masaoka stage I tumors, complete surgical resection is sufficient therapy and overall 5-year survival is 90% to 100%[15,26] The role of adjuvant radiotherapy for stage II tumors is controversial. The overall survival of Masaoka stage II patients is more than 80%, so a survival advantage for radiation in this group has been difficult to demonstrate.[27,28] There is general agreement that radiation therapy should be considered for patients with stage II disease after incomplete resection. Tumors stage III or higher and tumors that are greater than 4 cm in largest dimension may be best served by multimodality therapy.[9,29] At our institution, we typically use induction chemotherapy followed by surgery and then radiotherapy for advanced stage thymomas and thymic carcinomas. In a study of 22 patients with advanced thymomas (11 stage III, 10 stage IVa, 1 stage IVb, no thymic carcinomas) undergoing this approach to therapy, 76% of patients were able to achieve complete surgical resection. With a median follow-up of 50 months, the overall 5-year survival rate was 95%.[9] Locally advanced tumors may require resection of the superior vena cava, the innominate vein, part of the aorta, the pericardium, or 1 phrenic nerve. Bilateral phrenic nerve division should be avoided. Even in cases with isolated pleural metastases (stage IVa), if a complete resection is possible, patients can achieve long-term survival. Local recurrence and limited pleural recurrence can also be treated surgically with good outcomes, provided that complete excision is technically possible.[30] Goals for surgical resection should emphasize an R0, complete resection. Debulking operations are associated with lower overall survival and consideration should be given to alternative therapies.[8]

Germ Cell Tumors

Primary mediastinal GCTs compose 15% of anterior mediastinal masses in adults.[31] They are believed to arise from primitive germ cells that fail to migrate during embryogenesis. Testicular GCTs are far more common, comprising 95% to 98% of all GCTs in men. Extragonadal GCTs are split roughly equally between retroperitoneal and mediastinal primaries.[32] Both testicular and retroperitoneal GCTs may metastasize to the mediastinum. Therefore, the diagnosis of a mediastinal GCT should trigger a search for an extrathoracic primary. Primary mediastinal GCTs have a peak age of incidence in the third decade of life.[3,31] Mediastinal GCTs are divided into 3 cell types: mature teratomas, seminomas, and nonseminomatous GCTs. Whereas mature teratomas occur with equal frequency between men and women, malignant GCTs are much more common in men (>90%).[1]

Teratoma

Mature mediastinal teratoma is the most common mediastinal GCT.[31] Teratomas contain tissue from at least 2 of the 3 primitive germ layers. Ectodermal tissues include skin, sweat glands, hair, and toothlike structures. Mesodermal tissues include fat, cartilage, bone, and smooth muscle. Endodermal tissues include respiratory and intestinal epithelium and pancreatic tissue. Mature teratomas are almost always benign. If a teratoma contains fetal tissue, it is considered immature.[33] Immature teratomas have greater malignant potential and may be better treated with neoadjuvant chemotherapy followed by surgery.[34]

Many patients with mature teratomas are asymptomatic. Cough, chest pain, or dyspnea may occur as a result of local growth of the mass. The expectoration of hair (trichoptysis) occurs in about 5% of patients and is pathognomonic for teratoma.[35,36] Chest radiograph typically demonstrates a well-circumscribed mass. Calcification is seen about a quarter of the time, from a calcified tumor wall, bone, teeth, or nonspecific tissues.[36] CT shows a well-circumscribed, heterogeneous mass with varying amounts of soft tissue, fat, fluid, and calcium.

With a CT scan suggestive of teratoma, surgical resection without biopsy can proceed if there is no evidence of invasion of other structures. Complete surgical resection is curative with low rates of recurrence.[31,35]

Seminoma

Seminomas compose 25% to 40% of primary malignant mediastinal GCTs. The peak incidence is in the third decade of life and greater than 90% occur in men.[31,35,37,38] Most patients are symptomatic at presentation. Substernal chest pain, dyspnea, and cough are the most common presenting symptoms. Gynecomastia and superior vena cava syndrome may also accompany seminomas. Because gonadal seminomas may metastasize to the mediastinum, all patients with mediastinal seminoma should undergo a thorough lymph node and gonadal examination. Approximately 10% of patients with seminoma may have an increased beta-hCG level, but never an increased AFP level.[3] On CT scan, they are large, lobulated, well-circumscribed masses with relatively homogeneous attenuation.[36] The histology is essentially the same as gonadal seminomas. If any other germ cell types are present, the tumor is classified as a mixed GCT and is treated like a nonseminomatous GCT.[39] Metastatic disease is common at the time of presentation.[32]

Seminomas are highly sensitive to both chemotherapy and radiation. Chemotherapy may result in better progression-free survival than radiation therapy and is used more often as primary therapy, with an overall 5-year survival greater than 80%.[40] Treatment of residual masses following chemotherapy is controversial. Observation, radiotherapy, and surgery are all reasonable options, but none has clearly been shown to be superior.[41]

Nonseminomatous GCTs

Nonseminomatous GCTs comprise a heterogeneous group of histologies that include yolk sac tumor, choriocarcinoma, embryonal carcinoma, and mixed GCTs. Like seminomas, they occur predominantly in men and have a peak incidence in the third and fourth decades of life.[42] In addition to local symptoms of chest pain, dyspnea, cough, and superior vena cava syndrome, nonseminomatous GCTs are more likely to present with systemic symptoms of fever, chills, and weight loss. Gynecomastia may accompany beta-hCG secreting tumors. Kleinfelter syndrome may be observed in 20% of patients.[3] Most patients have an increased AFP level and many have an increased beta-hCG level.[31] The combination of an anterior mediastinal mass in a young man with an increased AFP level is so characteristic of a nonseminomatous GCT that some oncologists are willing to begin chemotherapy in this setting without a tissue diagnosis. Chemotherapy is the standard primary treatment, but fewer than half of patients have normalization of tumor markers following chemotherapy.[32] Whenever possible, complete surgical resection of residual tumor should be attempted after chemotherapy.[43,44] If viable tumor is identified in surgical specimens, additional chemotherapy is recommended. Nonseminomatous GCTs in the mediastinum carry a worse prognosis than retroperitoneal nonseminomatous GCTs. Even with multimodality therapy, the overall 5-year survival is only 40% to 60%.[32,45]

Thyroid

Substernal goiter is found in 3% to 20% of all operations for goiter.[46] Most are asymptomatic, but some patients may present with compression of the airway, dysphagia, hoarseness, or superior vena cava syndrome.[3] If a substernal goiter is suspected, iodinated contrast should be avoided because of the risk of iodine-induced hyperthyroidism and possible delay of radioiodine scanning. Radioactive iodine ablation has a low success rate for substernal goiter, therefore total thyroidectomy is the treatment of choice. The entire gland can be removed via a cervical approach in more than 95% of patients.[46] The surgery team should be aware of tracheomalacia associated with large goiters and the possibility of airway compromise (**Fig. 4**). Upwards of 10% of patients are not able to be extubated immediately postoperatively secondary to this effect. Informed surgical consent should contain a section on the possibility of tracheostomy.

Parathyroid

Ectopic parathyroid adenomas in the mediastinum are a common cause of failed operations for hyperparathyroidism. In 1 series of 285 patients with hyperparathyroidism, 20/53 (38%) of the reoperations had mediastinal parathyroid tumors. Eighty-one percent of the mediastinal parathyroids were in the anterior mediastinum and 19% were in the posterior mediastinum. Eighty-eight percent were removed via cervical incision.[47] Sestamibi scan is particularly helpful for identifying these ectopic adenomas.

Lymphoma

Most patients with mediastinal lymphoma have systemic disease and only 10% of patients have primary mediastinal lymphoma. The most common types of mediastinal lymphoma are Hodgkin disease, large B-cell lymphoma, and lymphoblastic lymphoma.[1,3,37] FNA is typically not sufficient for flow cytometry. Thus, the primary

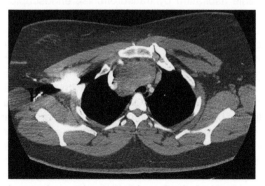

Fig. 4. CT scan of a large substernal goiter with tracheal compression.

role of the surgeon is for tissue diagnosis when core needle biopsy is not possible or is not sufficient for flow cytometry.

MIDDLE MEDIASTINUM

Lymphoma, granulomatous disease, mediastinal cysts, and tracheal tumors are the most common masses in the middle mediastinal. Aside from lymphoma, true tumors of the middle mediastinum are rare. Airway compression and dysphagia are the most common presenting symptoms.

Mediastinal Cysts

Mediastinal cysts are true cysts with fluid-filled, cell-lined sacs. They make up 12% to 25% of all mediastinal masses.[2,48,49] Although cysts may be found in any compartment of the mediastinum, they are most commonly found in the middle mediastinum. Most mediastinal cysts are asymptomatic in adults, but are more likely to be symptomatic in children.[49] A plain radiograph can often make the diagnosis, but CT scan should be obtained to better define the extent of the lesion. Cysts are usually distinguishable from solid tumors on CT scan.[5] CT typically demonstrates a round, well-demarcated, fluid-filled mass. The wall may or may not have calcifications. Some tumors (thymomas, GCTs) can undergo cystic degeneration and may be difficult to distinguish from a cyst. In addition, if a cyst contains nonserous fluid, it may appear solid on CT. In these cases, MRI may be helpful, demonstrating increased signal intensity on T2-weighted MRI.[5] Historically, surgeons have advocated resection of all bronchogenic cysts because up to 72% of these patients may become symptomatic or develop complications, at which time resection may be more difficult.[50] However, we have found that most asymptomatic cysts may be observed. Specific types of cysts are now described.

Enterogenous and bronchogenic cysts both develop as outgrowths from the primitive foregut in the fourth to eighth week of gestation.[51] Bronchogenic cysts compose 40% to 50% of mediastinal cysts.[48,49] They are lined by ciliated columnar epithelium and may contain bronchial glands and mucoid material. Cartilage is often found in the cyst wall. Forty percent of patients are symptomatic at presentation with chest pain, cough, and fever being the most common symptoms.[48] Most bronchogenic cysts are not in communication with the tracheobronchial tree and are homogeneous. However, if a communication or infection develops, an air-fluid level may be seen.[52] The diagnosis is often made radiologically. However, if a more definitive diagnosis is necessary, a needle aspiration by transbronchial, endoscopic, or percutaneous methods could be obtained.[53] Endobronchial ultrasound has also been reported for therapeutic aspiration and follow-up of a bronchogenic cyst.[54] Although rare, esophageal duplication cysts are the second most common enteric duplication cysts after ileal duplication cysts.[55] The cysts are lined by squamous or alimentary tract epithelium. They may contain gastric or pancreatic tissue. Symptoms are similar to bronchogenic cysts, but patients are more likely to present with dysphagia. Gastric mucosa may cause hemorrhage or perforation. The CT appearance is similar to bronchogenic cysts, but the wall may be thicker and more often calcified. Patients with possible esophageal duplication cysts should undergo barium swallow and endoscopy to determine communication with the lumen of the esophagus when symptomatic. Endoscopic ultrasound is accurate for the diagnosis of esophageal duplication cysts and is being used more frequently for their treatment. Endoscopic treatment via aspiration or resection of the cyst wall has been reported.[53,56]

Pericardial cysts are lined by mesothelium and are connected to the pericardium, although usually not in communication with the pericardial space. Most occur at the right cardiophrenic angle.[5] They are usually asymptomatic and present later in middle age, and are often found incidentally on echocardiography.[57] On CT, they are well circumscribed, round or teardrop shaped with homogeneous fluid. These cysts are usually observed if asymptomatic.

If there is a solid component or if the diagnosis is in doubt, mediastinal cysts may be aspirated. This often relieves any local symptoms as well. Depending on the location of the cyst, needle aspiration may be performed via a percutaneous, transbronchial, or transesophageal approach.[53,54] There is a chance of infecting a previously sterile cyst with aspiration, and most cysts can be removed thoracoscopically with low morbidity and minimal chance of recurrence.[58] Thus, in most cases, it may be more prudent to simply resect the cyst than risk infecting it with transbronchial or transesophageal aspiration.

POSTERIOR MEDIASTINUM

In the posterior mediastinum, neurogenic tumors and esophageal tumors are the most common masses.[2] Neuroenteric cysts are rare foregut malformations that contain both enteric and nerve tissue that are also found in the posterior mediastinum.[59] Neurogenic tumors constitute 75% of primary tumors in the posterior mediastinum.[2,60] Most arise from the spinal nerve roots or sympathetic chain and are located in the paravertebral sulcus. Most tumors in the posterior mediastinum are asymptomatic, but they may cause neuralgia or present with Horner syndrome from sympathetic ganglion involvement depending on location.[60,61] Neurogenic tumors are benign in 70% to 80% of cases.[2,60]

Neurogenic tumors have a characteristic appearance depending on their histology. MRI does not typically add much diagnostic information beyond CT, but may be of value in planning surgery, particularly for determining spinal cord involvement of neurogenic tumors.[62] *Meta*-Iodobenzylguanidine (MIBG) scans can help localize neuroblastomas and catecholamine-secreting paragangliomas.[63] Urine metanephrines and catecholamines should be measured in patients with paragangliomas who have symptoms or radiographic appearance suspicious for catecholamine-secreting tumor.

Nerve Sheath Tumors

Nerve sheath tumors compose 40% to 65% of neurogenic tumors in the chest.[1] Approximately 75% of these nerve sheath tumors are schwannomas (neurilemmomas) and 25% are neurofibromas. Whereas schwannomas are firm and encapsulated, neurofibromas are soft and nonencapsulated, although they may have a pseudocapsule; 10% to 30% of neurofibromas occur in association with neurofibromatosis. These are more likely to be multiple.[64] Malignant nerve sheath tumors are rare. They include malignant schwannomas, malignant neurofibromas, and neurogenic fibrosarcomas. Symptoms of pain and neurologic deficit are more common among malignant tumors. Approximately half of malignant nerve sheath tumors arise in the setting of neurofibromatosis.[65] Nerve sheath tumors may also grow outward and present as a chest wall mass.

On CT scan, nerve sheath tumors are typically round and well circumscribed. They grow into the intervertebral foramen and take on a dumbbell shape. MRI is helpful to evaluate intraspinal extension.[62] Nerve sheath tumors have increased signal intensity on T2-weighted MRI (**Fig. 5**). Traditionally, resection of all nerve sheath tumors has been recommended to exclude malignancy. However, the incidence of malignant

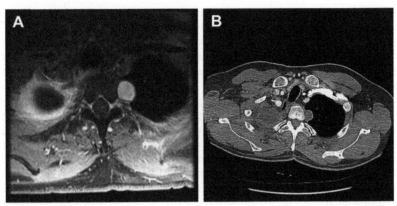

Fig. 5. MRI (*A*) and corresponding CT image (*B*) of an apical neurofibroma. The MRI shows increased signal intensity on a T2-weighted image.

nerve sheath tumor is so low that we recommend observation of small tumors without any high-risk features (symptoms, size >5 cm, previously irradiated field, evidence of invasion on CT or MRI).[65]

When necessary, benign nerve sheath tumors can be resected thoracoscopically in more than 90% of cases.[66,67] Dumbbell tumors may be removed with a combined open neurosurgical approach for the spinal component and a thoracosocpic approach for the thoracic component. Horner syndrome, sympathectomy, and paraplegia are possible complications, but all of these usually improve with time. A more radical resection, often including a chest wall resection, is the treatment of choice for malignant nerve sheath tumors. Adjuvant chemotherapy and radiation may also be of value in this setting.[65]

Ganglion Tumors

Autonomic ganglion tumors in the mediastinum usually occur in the sympathetic ganglia, but may occasionally occur in the parasympathetic ganglia. These tumors arise from nerve cells rather than the nerve sheaths.[63] They are primarily pediatric tumors, with two-thirds occurring in patients less than 20 years of age. Unlike nerve sheath tumors, most ganglion tumors are malignant.[61,68] On imaging, they are typically oblong-shaped, well-circumscribed, large masses that occur along the anterolateral border of the spine. On CT scan, they are more likely to have calcifications than nerve sheath tumors.[69]

Ganglioneuromas are the most common benign ganglion tumors in the mediastinum. They are well-differentiated tumors and most are asymptomatic.[70] They are treated by complete surgical resection.

Neuroblastomas are principally pediatric tumors. Most are diagnosed before 2 years age and the tumor is rare after the age of 10 years. Overall, it is the most common extracranial solid cancer in children, accounting for 6% to 10% of all childhood cancers and 15% of childhood cancer mortality in the United States.[71] Neuroblastomas are nonencapsulated and have small round cells on histology. They are associated with amplification of the *MYCN* oncogene. The tumors are highly aggressive and are frequently metastatic at presentation. Up to 30% of neuroblastomas arise in the mediastinum. In addition to local symptoms, patients may present with fatigue, weight loss, or fever. Neuroblastomas are sometimes associated with paraneoplastic syndromes, including severe diarrhea from vasoactive intestinal peptide and opsomyoclonus. On CT scan 80% of neuroblastomas show calcification. MIBG scanning is helpful for demonstrating the extent of disease and identifying metastatic disease.[63] Complete surgical resection is the treatment of choice for early stage tumors. Although somewhat controversial, neoadjuvant therapy has been shown to increase the likelihood of complete excision for more advanced tumors.[71] Ganglioneuroblastomas are rare tumors that have features of both ganglioneuromas and neuroblastomas. They are staged similarly to neuroblastomas and prognosis depends on histology.[63]

CHEST WALL TUMORS

Tumors of the chest wall can be either primary or secondary. The secondary tumors are caused by either local invasion (from breast, lung, or pleural cancers) or distant metastases. Primary chest wall tumors are rare, but include a wide variety of benign and malignant histologies (**Table 3**). Among primary tumors of the chest wall, roughly half are benign and half are malignant.[72]

History

Chest wall resections were exceedingly rare until the twentieth century, when the development of anesthesia, asepsis, and positive pressure ventilation allowed chest

Table 3 Primary chest wall tumors	
Soft Tissue	
Benign	Lipoma
	Elastofibroma
	Neurofibroma
	Lymphangioma
	Hemangioma
	Hamartoma
Desmoid	
Malignant	Malignant fibrous histiocytoma
	Liposarcoma
	Leiomyosarcoma
	Spindle cell sarcoma
	Angiosarcoma
	Synovial cell sarcoma
	Fibrosarcoma
	Rhabdomyosarcoma
	Undifferentiated sarcoma
	Lymphoma
Bone and Cartilage	
Benign	Fibrous dysplasia
	Enchondroma
	Osteochondroma
	Aneurysmal bone cyst
	Osteoid osteoma
	Osteoblastoma
	Eosinophilic granuloma
	Giant cell tumor
Malignant	Chondrosarcoma
	Osteosarcoma
	Ewing sarcoma
	Primitive neuroectodermal tumor
	Solitary plasmacytoma

wall resections to be performed safely. In 1887, Joseph O'Dwyer developed a steel apparatus that could be intubated into the larynx and attached to a bellows previously developed by George Fell to deliver positive pressure ventilation. A decade later, F.W. Parham reported using the device in a series of chest wall resections. The following passage from his address to the Southern Surgical Association in 1887 underscores the technical challenges posed by such operations:

> I operated in the Charity Hospital ... for a sarcoma of the thoracic wall requiring the resection of several inches of the third, fourth, and fifth ribs .... A rent of five inches was made, which permitted easily the thrusting of the whole hand into the pleural cavity. Suddenly was presented to our anxious view one of the most startling clinical pictures that the surgeon can ever be called upon to witness. At such a sight the stoutest heart will quaver.

In Parham's review of the world literature at the time, he reported a perioperative mortality rate of 30%.[73] Since that time, advances in anesthesia and perioperative care have improved the mortality for thoracic surgery. In addition, the development of reconstructive techniques has helped decrease the long-term morbidity of chest wall resection. Today, surgery is the main therapy for most primary chest wall malignancies and postoperative mortality should approach zero. Advances in imaging and adjuvant therapy continue to improve the diagnosis and treatment of these rare tumors.

Chest Wall Anatomy

A thorough understanding of the structure and function of the chest wall is critical to the evaluation and treatment of chest wall tumors. The chest wall provides a semi-rigid cage that protects the thoracic viscera but allows for respiratory movement.[74] The bony frame is formed by the ribs, vertebral bodies, and sternum. Normally, there are 12 paired ribs on each side. The first 7 are referred to as true ribs, whereas the bottom 5 are referred to as false ribs. Anteriorly, the true ribs are attached to the costal cartilage of the sternum. The 8th to 10th ribs connect to the costal cartilage of the seventh rib. The bottom 2 ribs are unattached anteriorly and are referred to as floating ribs.

The structure of the chest wall facilitates respiratory mechanics, allowing effective ventilation. The curvature of the lower ribs causes a bucket handle type of movement with inspiration, allowing the ribs to move laterally and cephalad and helping the lower chest to expand in volume. The external intercostals contribute to the lateral and cephalad retraction of the ribs during inspiration, whereas the internal and innermost intercostals contribute expiratory force.

The muscles of the chest wall serve a variety of functions. The accessory muscles of respiration include the scalenes, trapezius, pectoralis minor, rhomboids, and serratus. The scapula and clavicle form the pectoral girdle, which connects the upper extremity to the axial skeleton. The rhomboids and trapezius retract the pectoral girdle, whereas the serratus anterior and pectoralis minor protract (push) the pectoral girdle. The supraspinatus, pectoralis major, latissimus dorsi, teres major, teres minor, subscapularis, and infraspinatus all aid in movement of the upper extremity. A thorough understanding of the blood supply of these muscles is critical for chest wall resections because they may be used for flap coverage and reconstruction.

General Approach to Chest Wall Tumors

Most tumors of the chest wall present either as an enlarging, asymptomatic mass or with pain. Bony and cartilaginous tumors are often identified incidentally on imaging. The presence of pain is more common with malignant lesions. Many tumors, particularly cartilaginous tumors, have a characteristic radiologic appearance.[75] If a suspicious osseous lesion is seen on routine chest radiograph, a dedicated, lower voltage bone radiograph may better delineate the abnormality. CT scan is usually necessary to identify the extent of the lesion and aid in planning possible resection. MRI is helpful for determining disc space or neural involvement.[76] PET is not a routine part of the evaluation of chest wall tumors, but there are some data that PET may be more accurate than CT scan for determining the extent of large tumors.[77] The use of ultrasound to mark the edges of a tumor has also been shown to help in obtaining negative surgical margins.[78]

Historically, incisional biopsy has often been performed for diagnosis; however, at our institution, we have found that FNA or core needle biopsy is preferable and usually sufficient for diagnosis with a skilled cytopathologist.[79,80] The biopsy track should be within the planned excision site whenever possible. Therefore, biopsy is preferably performed at the treating center rather than the referring center. Excisional biopsy may be performed for benign-appearing tumors less than 2 cm involving only 1 rib. If malignancy is found, then a wider excision may be performed. For malignant or large tumors, a multidisciplinary approach is valuable for planning neoadjuvant therapy, reconstruction, and adjuvant therapy.

Soft Tissue Tumors

Benign

Deep chest wall lipomas can be difficult to distinguish from liposarcoma or other sarcomas by physical examination. On CT, lipomas are typically homogeneous and do not enhance with intravenous contrast, whereas liposarcomas have heterogeneous enhancement and tend to be larger. They both have high signal intensity on T2-weighted MRI.[81]

Elastofibromas are benign tumors that classically occur in the subscapular region. They have a female predominance with a peak incidence in the 40- to 70-year-old age range. These tumors have a characteristic layered appearance on CT and exhibit mild enhancement with intravenous contrast.[82] Local excision is curative.

Other benign lesions found in the soft tissue of the chest wall include neurofibroma, lymphangioma, and hamartoma.

Desmoid

Desmoid tumors are rare tumors that do not metastasize but can be difficult to treat because of their locally aggressive nature and propensity for local recurrence. They are often associated with familial adenomatous polyposis. Most desmoids tumors occur in the abdominal wall, but the chest wall and shoulder girdle are common sites for extra-abdominal disease.[83] The peak incidence is in the second and third decades of life. On CT and MRI, desmoid tumors have a variable nondescript appearance depending on the amount of collagen content, but generally have similar enhancement to muscle.[76]

Local control can be difficult, particularly in the chest. The recurrence rate for chest wall desmoids tumors is 25% to 75%.[83–85] Wide margins are critical because of the high incidence of microscopic positive margins. In a series of 53 patients with desmoids tumors of the chest wall, 7 (13%) had positive margins. The local recurrence rate was 89% for those with positive margins, compared with 18% for those with negative margins.[84] Chemotherapy using a doxorubicin-based regimen may be of benefit in the adjuvant setting. Antiestrogens, such as tamoxifen have also been used.[86] Radiation therapy is typically used for unresectable disease, for locally recurrent disease, or to treat positive margins, but its effectiveness remains uncertain.

Soft tissue sarcomas

Soft tissue sarcomas of the chest come in a wide range of histologies, including malignant fibrous histiocytoma (MFH), angiosarcoma, leiomyosarcoma, synovial cell sarcoma, spindle cell, liposarcoma, and undifferentiated sarcomas. These tumors can arise either de novo or in the setting of previous radiation therapy. On CT, they usually have a heterogeneous appearance with varying levels of enhancement with intravenous contrast.[87] Depending on the histology, sarcomas demonstrate varying degrees of calcification on CT scan.[88] The diagnosis cannot be made radiologically and therefore requires tissue for confirmation. Normally a core biopsy is sufficient.

The mainstay of therapy for soft tissue sarcomas is surgical resection with wide margins. A 2-cm margin is recommended for low-grade sarcomas, and a 4-cm margin with resection of a rib above and below the tumor is recommended for high-grade sarcomas.[79] Published series report 5-year survival rates with a wide range (50%–80%), reflecting the heterogeneity of these tumors.[79,89–92] Margin status, grade of tumor, and histology have all been shown to be associated with survival.[93,94] Because chest wall sarcomas are rare, the use of adjuvant therapies for these lesions has largely been extrapolated from experience with extremity sarcomas. For large tumors or if there is any question about the resectability of a tumor, a multidisciplinary approach with neoadjuvant therapy should be considered. If it can be done safely, reoperation should also be performed for local recurrences. Wouters and colleagues[95] reported a 5-year survival rate of 50% following reoperation for recurrent chest wall sarcoma without a significantly increased risk of perioperative complications.

Cartilage and Bone

Metastatic tumors of the bones and cartilage of the chest wall are far more common than primary tumors. Primary tumors are equally likely to be benign or malignant. Tumors arising in the sternum are more likely to be malignant.[76,96]

Benign Tumors

Fibrous dysplasia (FD) is the most common benign tumor of the ribs, accounting for 30% of benign chest wall tumors.[96] FD is not a true neoplasm, but is a tumor that occurs because of the failure of osteoblasts to undergo normal maturation. The marrow is instead replaced by immature bone and fibrous stroma. FD is slow growing and typically asymptomatic at presentation, although may present with pathologic fracture or local pain. In 75% of patients FD is monostotic, affecting 1 rib; in 25% it is polyostotic, affecting multiple ribs or other bones. Monostotic FD most commonly affects the second rib. When polyostotic FD is associated with café-au-lait macules and endocrine abnormalities, it is known as McCune-Albright syndrome.[97] The diagnosis of FD is usually made radiologically and these lesions do not require therapy unless symptomatic.

Osteochondroma and enchondroma are the next most common benign tumors of thoracic bones and cartilage, but each composes less than 10% of primary chest wall tumors.[96,98] They have a peak incidence in the second decade of life. Osteochondromas arise from the cortex of bone and are characterized by a cartilaginous covering. Fifteen percent of osteochondromas occur in the setting of multiple hereditary exostoses. In the chest, osteochondromas are most commonly found at the costochondral junction. The risk of malignant degeneration to chondrosarcoma is related to the thickness of the cartilaginous cap. Caps greater than 2 cm thick are suspicious for carcinoma.[81,96] Enchondromas are cartilaginous tumors that arise from the medullary cavity. They have a lobulated appearance with distinct borders. In the chest, enchondromas typically occur in the anterior portions of the ribs.

Aneurysmal bone cysts (ABCs) are osteolytic lesions with blood-filled cystic spaces. ABCs are often associated with abnormal bone. They are sometimes preceded by trauma or may be found in the setting of an underlying bone tumor such as osteoblastoma. In the chest, they are typically located in the lateral and posterior ribs. Surgery is the mainstay of treatment with cure rates of 70% to 90%.[99] ABCs do not metastasize, but radiation therapy is occasionally used for local control in the setting of locally aggressive or recurrent tumors.

Langerhans cell histiocytosis (LCH), formerly known as histiocytosis X, can affect many different types of tissue, but commonly affects bone. Bony involvement can be monostotic or polyostotic.[100] Eosinophilic granuloma is a form of LCH that is isolated to the bone. Most forms of LCH are not treated surgically, but isolated eosinophilic granuloma can be treated with resection or curettage with good results. Most eosinophilic granulomas are monostotic and affect children less than 15 years of age. Solitary eosinophilic granulomas involve the ribs in 9% to 15% of patients. The destructive lytic appearance may resemble Ewing sarcoma, particularly if there is a significant soft tissue component. Osteoid osteoma is the most common benign bone tumor overall, accounting for 10% to 20% of benign bone tumors in the body.[101] However, it is rare in the ribs and accounts for only 1% of primary rib tumors. It is characterized by a nidus of osteoid tissue surrounded by a rim of reactive sclerotic bone. In the chest, it usually presents with pain, particularly at night. Most tumors occur in the posterior rib and have a characteristic appearance on bone scan, called the doubled density sign.[96] Osteoblastoma has many similarities to osteoid osteoma and was known formerly as giant osteoid osteoma. It is also rare in the ribs. Lesions are typically larger than osteoid osteoma and do not have a central nidus. Although osteoblastomas are benign, they may be locally aggressive with potential for local recurrence, thus resection of all affected bone is the preferred treatment.[102] Giant cell tumors occur rarely in the ribs, with a peak incidence in the third and fourth decades of life. Although considered benign, they can be locally aggressive. Wide local excision is recommended.[96,103]

Malignant

Chondrosarcoma

Chondrosarcoma is the most common primary malignant tumor of the chest wall. They most commonly occur along the costochondral junction. The age of presentation has 2 peaks: 1 in the second decade of life and the other in the fifth decade of life.[87] There is a slight male predominance.[88] Most patients present with a large mass, which may or may not be accompanied by pain. Depending on the degree of differentiation and invasion, tumors can have a wide range of appearance on imaging. CT demonstrates areas of calcification in the chondroid matrix (**Fig. 6**). Surgery with wide margins is the primary mode of treatment. Incomplete resection is associated with decreased survival. In 1 series of 106 patients with chest wall chondrosarcoma, patients who underwent surgery with wide margins had a 10-year survival rate of 92%, compared with 47% for incomplete resection. The local recurrence rates were 4% and 73%, respectively.[104] Radiation therapy has been shown to help with local control for recurrent or incompletely resected disease. Chemotherapy has not yet been shown to provide significant benefit, except possibly for mesenchymal or dedifferentiated subtypes.[105]

Osteosarcoma

Although osteosarcoma is the most common malignant bone tumor throughout the body, it is rare in the chest wall. Only 1% to 3% of osteosarcomas involve the chest wall.[106,107] The peak incidence is in the second decade of life. Like the other malignant

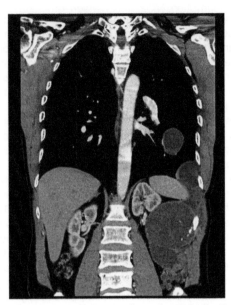

Fig. 6. CT scan of a chondrosarcoma originating from the 10th rib. Note the extensive intra-abdominal as well as intrathoracic component of the tumor.

bony tumors of the chest wall, most patients present with a painful mass. On CT, there is typically a large mass that is heterogeneous with areas of bony destruction (**Fig. 7**). Because of the poor results from single modality therapy for osteosarcomas of the chest wall, these tumors are typically treated with neoadjuvant chemotherapy followed by surgery. As with the other sarcomas, clear margins are associated with improved survival. Osteosarcomas are not very radiosensitive, but radiation therapy has been used for tumors with inadequate resection. The overall survival, even with neoadjuvant therapy, is 15% to 27% at 5 years compared with 65% to 75% for extremity osteosarcomas.[107]

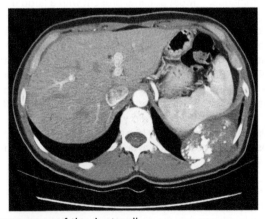

Fig. 7. Primary osteosarcoma of the chest wall.

Ewing sarcoma and primary neuroectodermal tumors

The Ewing sarcoma family of tumors includes Ewing sarcoma and primitive neuroectodermal tumor (PNET). These tumors harbor the same chromosomal translocation t(11;22) and are believed to arise from primitive cells of the neural crest.[108] PNETs that arise in the chest are also known as Askin tumors.[109] Ewing sarcoma/PNET tumors typically occur in the first 2 decades of life and are the most common tumor of the chest wall in children and young adults.[110] In the chest, Ewing sarcoma most commonly affects the ribs, but may arise in the paravertebral region or occasionally in the soft tissue. Most patients have pain as a presenting symptom. CT scan typically shows a large ill-defined tumor with cystic degeneration with soft tissue extension. Tumors usually have increased signal intensity on T1-weighted MRI and intermediate intensity on T2-weighted images.[87,109] However, larger tumors have heterogeneous intensity. Retrospective analysis from an intergroup study found that patients with Ewing sarcoma of the rib were more likely to undergo complete resection and avoid radiation therapy if chemotherapy was given before surgery.[111,112] Therefore, it is recommended that most patients with Ewing sarcoma undergo multimodality therapy. Radiation therapy has been shown to provide good local control when complete resection is not possible, but has significant cardiopulmonary toxicities in the chest and also has oncogenic potential in such a young patient population.[113] Five-year survival is greater than 60% with chemotherapy and surgery.[111]

Reconstruction of the Chest Wall

Reconstruction of the chest wall can be complex and often requires working with a plastic surgery team. The ideal reconstruction provides protection to the thoracic viscera and preserves respiratory mechanics with a good cosmetic outcome. For posterior rib defects, the scapula may provide adequate coverage and stabilization. For lateral and anterior defects greater than 5 cm in diameter, a synthetic material is used to provide a frame, which is covered by vascularized tissue. Polypropylene and polytetrafluoroethylene are the most commonly used synthetic meshes. In cases where rigidity is required, we typically use methyl methacrylate sandwiched between 2 pieces of Marlex mesh. This should then be covered with a vascularized tissue flap. A variety of pedicled and free muscle flaps have been described for chest wall reconstruction. Omental flaps may also be used, but require a laparotomy and may lead to hernia formation.[114]

REFERENCES

1. Duwe BV, Sterman DH, Musani AI. Tumors of the mediastinum. Chest 2005;128: 2893.
2. Davis RD Jr, Oldham HN Jr, Sabiston DC Jr. Primary cysts and neoplasms of the mediastinum: recent changes in clinical presentation, methods of diagnosis, management, and results. Ann Thorac Surg 1987;44:229.
3. Strollo DC, Rosado de Christenson ML, Jett JR. Primary mediastinal tumors. Part 1: tumors of the anterior mediastinum. Chest 1997;112:511.
4. Basaria S, Salvatori R. Images in clinical medicine. Pemberton's sign. N Engl J Med 2004;350:1338.
5. Jeung MY, Gasser B, Gangi A, et al. Imaging of cystic masses of the mediastinum. Radiographics 2002;22(Spec No):S79.
6. Kebebew E, Arici C, Duh QY, et al. Localization and reoperation results for persistent and recurrent parathyroid carcinoma. Arch Surg 2001;136:878.

7. Bagga S, Bloch EM. Imaging of an invasive malignant thymoma on PET scan: CT and histopathologic correlation. Clin Nucl Med 2006;31:614.

8. Kaiser LR. Surgical treatment of thymic epithelial neoplasms. Hematol Oncol Clin North Am 2008;22:475.

9. Kim ES, Putnam JB, Komaki R, et al. Phase II study of a multidisciplinary approach with induction chemotherapy, followed by surgical resection, radiation therapy, and consolidation chemotherapy for unresectable malignant thymomas: final report. Lung Cancer 2004;44:369.

10. Assaad MW, Pantanowitz L, Otis CN. Diagnostic accuracy of image-guided percutaneous fine needle aspiration biopsy of the mediastinum. Diagn Cytopathol 2007;35:705.

11. Annessi V, Paci M, Ferrari G, et al. Ultrasonically guided biopsy of anterior mediastinal masses. Interact Cardiovasc Thorac Surg 2003;2:319.

12. Mullen B, Richardson JD. Primary anterior mediastinal tumors in children and adults. Ann Thorac Surg 1986;42:338.

13. Tomaszek S, Wigle DA, Keshavjee S, et al. Thymomas: review of current clinical practice. Ann Thorac Surg 2009;87:1973.

14. Wilkins KB, Sheikh E, Green R, et al. Clinical and pathologic predictors of survival in patients with thymoma. Ann Surg 1999;230:562.

15. Falkson CB, Bezjak A, Darling G, et al. The management of thymoma: a systematic review and practice guideline. J Thorac Oncol 2009;4:911.

16. Drachman DB. Myasthenia gravis. N Engl J Med 1994;330:1797.

17. Blossom GB, Ernstoff RM, Howells GA, et al. Thymectomy for myasthenia gravis. Arch Surg 1993;128:855.

18. Buckingham JM, Howard FM Jr, Bernatz PE, et al. The value of thymectomy in myasthenia gravis: a computer-assisted matched study. Ann Surg 1976; 184:453.

19. Masaoka A, Monden Y, Nakahara K, et al. Follow-up study of thymomas with special reference to their clinical stages. Cancer 1981;48:2485.

20. Schneider PM, Fellbaum C, Fink U, et al. Prognostic importance of histomorphologic subclassification for epithelial thymic tumors. Ann Surg Oncol 1997; 4:46.

21. Travis WD. World Health Organization. International Agency for Research on Cancer. Pathology and genetics of tumours of the lung, pleura, thymus and heart. Lyon (France): IARC Press; 2004.

22. Rena O, Papalia E, Maggi G, et al. World Health Organization histologic classification: an independent prognostic factor in resected thymomas. Lung Cancer 2005;50:59.

23. Eng TY, Fuller CD, Jagirdar J, et al. Thymic carcinoma: state of the art review. Int J Radiat Oncol Biol Phys 2004;59:654.

24. Cardillo G, Treggiari S, Paul MA, et al. Primary neuroendocrine tumours of the thymus: a clinicopathologic and prognostic study in 19 patients. Eur J Cardiothorac Surg 2010;37(4):814–8.

25. Cheng YJ, Kao EL, Chou SH. Videothoracoscopic resection of stage II thymoma: prospective comparison of the results between thoracoscopy and open methods. Chest 2005;128:3010.

26. Davenport E, Malthaner RA. The role of surgery in the management of thymoma: a systematic review. Ann Thorac Surg 2008;86:673.

27. Ogawa K, Uno T, Toita T, et al. Postoperative radiotherapy for patients with completely resected thymoma: a multi-institutional, retrospective review of 103 patients. Cancer 2002;94:1405.

28. Rena O, Papalia E, Oliaro A, et al. Does adjuvant radiation therapy improve disease-free survival in completely resected Masaoka stage II thymoma? Eur J Cardiothorac Surg 2007;31:109.
29. Huang J, Rizk NP, Travis WD, et al. Feasibility of multimodality therapy including extended resections in stage IVA thymoma. J Thorac Cardiovasc Surg 2007; 134:1477.
30. Okumura M, Shiono H, Inoue M, et al. Outcome of surgical treatment for recurrent thymic epithelial tumors with reference to World Health Organization histologic classification system. J Surg Oncol 2007;95:40.
31. Nichols CR. Mediastinal germ cell tumors. Clinical features and biologic correlates. Chest 1991;99:472.
32. Bokemeyer C, Nichols CR, Droz JP, et al. Extragonadal germ cell tumors of the mediastinum and retroperitoneum: results from an international analysis. J Clin Oncol 2002;20:1864.
33. Moran CA, Suster S. Primary germ cell tumors of the mediastinum: I. Analysis of 322 cases with special emphasis on teratomatous lesions and a proposal for histopathologic classification and clinical staging. Cancer 1997;80:681.
34. Arai K, Ohta S, Suzuki M, et al. Primary immature mediastinal teratoma in adulthood. Eur J Surg Oncol 1997;23:64.
35. Lewis BD, Hurt RD, Payne WS, et al. Benign teratomas of the mediastinum. J Thorac Cardiovasc Surg 1983;86:727.
36. Drevelegas A, Palladas P, Scordalaki A. Mediastinal germ cell tumors: a radiologic-pathologic review. Eur Radiol 2001;11:1925.
37. Macchiarini P, Ostertag H. Uncommon primary mediastinal tumours. Lancet Oncol 2004;5:107.
38. Sakurai H, Asamura H, Suzuki K, et al. Management of primary malignant germ cell tumor of the mediastinum. Jpn J Clin Oncol 2004;34:386.
39. Moran CA, Suster S, Przygodzki RM, et al. Primary germ cell tumors of the mediastinum: II. Mediastinal seminomas–a clinicopathologic and immunohistochemical study of 120 cases. Cancer 1997;80:691.
40. Bokemeyer C, Droz JP, Horwich A, et al. Extragonadal seminoma: an international multicenter analysis of prognostic factors and long term treatment outcome. Cancer 2001;91:1394.
41. Puc HS, Heelan R, Mazumdar M, et al. Management of residual mass in advanced seminoma: results and recommendations from the Memorial Sloan-Kettering Cancer Center. J Clin Oncol 1996;14:454.
42. Moran CA, Suster S, Koss MN. Primary germ cell tumors of the mediastinum: III. Yolk sac tumor, embryonal carcinoma, choriocarcinoma, and combined nonteratomatous germ cell tumors of the mediastinum–a clinicopathologic and immunohistochemical study of 64 cases. Cancer 1997;80:699.
43. Vuky J, Bains M, Bacik J, et al. Role of postchemotherapy adjunctive surgery in the management of patients with nonseminoma arising from the mediastinum. J Clin Oncol 2001;19:682.
44. Walsh GL, Taylor GD, Nesbitt JC, et al. Intensive chemotherapy and radical resections for primary nonseminomatous mediastinal germ cell tumors. Ann Thorac Surg 2000;69:337.
45. Bukowski RM, Wolf M, Kulander BG, et al. Alternating combination chemotherapy in patients with extragonadal germ cell tumors. A Southwest Oncology Group study. Cancer 1993;71:2631.
46. Shen WT, Kebebew E, Duh QY, et al. Predictors of airway complications after thyroidectomy for substernal goiter. Arch Surg 2004;139:656.

47. Clark OH. Mediastinal parathyroid tumors. Arch Surg 1988;123:1096.
48. Takeda S, Miyoshi S, Minami M, et al. Clinical spectrum of mediastinal cysts. Chest 2003;124:125.
49. Strollo DC, Rosado-de-Christenson ML, Jett JR. Primary mediastinal tumors: part II. Tumors of the middle and posterior mediastinum. Chest 1997;112:1344.
50. Cioffi U, Bonavina L, De Simone M, et al. Presentation and surgical management of bronchogenic and esophageal duplication cysts in adults. Chest 1998;113: 1492.
51. Berrocal T, Madrid C, Novo S, et al. Congenital anomalies of the tracheobronchial tree, lung, and mediastinum: embryology, radiology, and pathology. Radiographics 2004;24:e17.
52. Kim Y, Lee KS, Yoo JH, et al. Middle mediastinal lesions: imaging findings and pathologic correlation. Eur J Radiol 2000;35:30.
53. Chen VK, Eloubeidi MA. Endoscopic ultrasound-guided fine-needle aspiration of intramural and extraintestinal mass lesions: diagnostic accuracy, complication assessment, and impact on management. Endoscopy 2005;37:984.
54. Galluccio G, Lucantoni G. Mediastinal bronchogenic cyst's recurrence treated with EBUS-FNA with a long-term follow-up. Eur J Cardiothorac Surg 2006;29:627.
55. Holcomb GW 3rd, Gheissari A, O'Neill JA Jr, et al. Surgical management of alimentary tract duplications. Ann Surg 1989;209:167.
56. Will U, Meyer F, Bosseckert H. Successful endoscopic treatment of an esophageal duplication cyst. Scand J Gastroenterol 2005;40:995.
57. Patel J, Park C, Michaels J, et al. Pericardial cyst: case reports and a literature review. Echocardiography 2004;21:269.
58. Hirose S, Clifton MS, Bratton B, et al. Thoracoscopic resection of foregut duplication cysts. J Laparoendosc Adv Surg Tech A 2006;16:526.
59. Setty H, Hegde KK, Narvekar VN. Neurenteric cyst of the posterior mediastinum. Australas Radiol 2005;49:151.
60. Davidson KG, Walbaum PR, McCormack RJ. Intrathoracic neural tumours. Thorax 1978;33:359.
61. Parish C. Complications of mediastinal neural tumours. Thorax 1971;26:392.
62. Tanaka O, Kiryu T, Hirose Y, et al. Neurogenic tumors of the mediastinum and chest wall: MR imaging appearance. J Thorac Imaging 2005;20:316.
63. Lonergan GJ, Schwab CM, Suarez ES, et al. Neuroblastoma, ganglioneuroblastoma, and ganglioneuroma: radiologic-pathologic correlation. Radiographics 2002;22:911.
64. Reed JC, Hallet KK, Feigin DS. Neural tumors of the thorax: subject review from the AFIP. Radiology 1978;126:9.
65. Ducatman BS, Scheithauer BW, Piepgras DG, et al. Malignant peripheral nerve sheath tumors. A clinicopathologic study of 120 cases. Cancer 1986;57:2006.
66. Kumar A, Kumar S, Aggarwal S, et al. Thoracoscopy: the preferred approach for the resection of selected posterior mediastinal tumors. J Laparoendosc Adv Surg Tech A 2002;12:345.
67. Liu HP, Yim AP, Wan J, et al. Thoracoscopic removal of intrathoracic neurogenic tumors: a combined Chinese experience. Ann Surg 2000;232:187.
68. Adam A, Hochholzer L. Ganglioneuroblastoma of the posterior mediastinum: a clinicopathologic review of 80 cases. Cancer 1981;47:373.
69. Kawashima A, Fishman EK, Kuhlman JE, et al. CT of posterior mediastinal masses. Radiographics 1991;11:1045.
70. Forsythe A, Volpe J, Muller R. Posterior mediastinal ganglioneuroma. Radiographics 2004;24:594.

71. Ishola TA, Chung DH. Neuroblastoma. Surg Oncol 2007;16:149.
72. Graeber GM, Snyder RJ, Fleming AW, et al. Initial and long-term results in the management of primary chest wall neoplasms. Ann Thorac Surg 1982;34:664.
73. Parham FW. Thoracic resection for tumors growing from the bony wall of the chest. New Orleans (LA): [sn]; 1899.
74. Pearson FG. Thoracic surgery. 2nd edition. New York: Churchill Livingstone; 2002.
75. Meyer CA, White CS. Cartilaginous disorders of the chest. Radiographics 1998; 18:1109.
76. Jeung MY, Gangi A, Gasser B, et al. Imaging of chest wall disorders. Radiographics 1999;19:617.
77. Petermann D, Allenbach G, Schmidt S, et al. Value of positron emission tomography in full-thickness chest wall resections for malignancies. Interact Cardiovasc Thorac Surg 2009;9:406.
78. Briccoli A, Galletti S, Salone M, et al. Ultrasonography is superior to computed tomography and magnetic resonance imaging in determining superficial resection margins of malignant chest wall tumors. J Ultrasound Med 2007;26:157.
79. Walsh GL, Davis BM, Swisher SG, et al. A single-institutional, multidisciplinary approach to primary sarcomas involving the chest wall requiring full-thickness resections. J Thorac Cardiovasc Surg 2001;121:48.
80. Goel A, Gupta SK, Dey P, et al. Cytologic spectrum of 227 fine-needle aspiration cases of chest-wall lesions. Diagn Cytopathol 2001;24:384.
81. Tateishi U, Gladish GW, Kusumoto M, et al. Chest wall tumors: radiologic findings and pathologic correlation: part 1. Benign tumors. Radiographics 2003; 23:1477.
82. Freixinet J, Rodriguez P, Hussein M, et al. Elastofibroma of the thoracic wall. Interact Cardiovasc Thorac Surg 2008;7:626.
83. Kabiri EH, Al Aziz S, El Maslout A, et al. Desmoid tumors of the chest wall. Eur J Cardiothorac Surg 2001;19:580.
84. Abbas AE, Deschamps C, Cassivi SD, et al. Chest-wall desmoid tumors: results of surgical intervention. Ann Thorac Surg 2004;78:1219.
85. Zisis C, Dountsis A, Nikolaides A, et al. Desmoid tumors of the chest wall. Asian Cardiovasc Thorac Ann 2006;14:359.
86. Ohashi T, Shigematsu N, Kameyama K, et al. Tamoxifen for recurrent desmoid tumor of the chest wall. Int J Clin Oncol 2006;11:150.
87. Tateishi U, Gladish GW, Kusumoto M, et al. Chest wall tumors: radiologic findings and pathologic correlation: part 2. Malignant tumors. Radiographics 2003;23:1491.
88. Gladish GW, Sabloff BM, Munden RF, et al. Primary thoracic sarcomas. Radiographics 2002;22:621.
89. Tsukushi S, Nishida Y, Sugiura H, et al. Soft tissue sarcomas of the chest wall. J Thorac Oncol 2009;4:834.
90. Burt M. Primary malignant tumors of the chest wall. The Memorial Sloan-Kettering Cancer Center experience. Chest Surg Clin N Am 1994;4:137.
91. Athanassiadi K, Kalavrouziotis G, Rondogianni D, et al. Primary chest wall tumors: early and long-term results of surgical treatment. Eur J Cardiothorac Surg 2001;19:589.
92. Hsu PK, Hsu HS, Lee HC, et al. Management of primary chest wall tumors: 14 years' clinical experience. J Chin Med Assoc 2006;69:377.
93. Gordon MS, Hajdu SI, Bains MS, et al. Soft tissue sarcomas of the chest wall. Results of surgical resection. J Thorac Cardiovasc Surg 1991;101:843.

94. Gross JL, Younes RN, Haddad FJ, et al. Soft-tissue sarcomas of the chest wall: prognostic factors. Chest 2005;127:902.
95. Wouters MW, van Geel AN, Nieuwenhuis L, et al. Outcome after surgical resections of recurrent chest wall sarcomas. J Clin Oncol 2008;26:5113.
96. Hughes EK, James SL, Butt S, et al. Benign primary tumours of the ribs. Clin Radiol 2006;61:314.
97. O'Connor B, Collins FJ. The management of chest wall resection in a patient with polyostotic fibrous dysplasia and respiratory failure. J Cardiothorac Vasc Anesth 2009;23:518.
98. Kim S, Lee S, Arsenault DA, et al. Pediatric rib lesions: a 13-year experience. J Pediatr Surg 2008;43:1781.
99. Mendenhall WM, Zlotecki RA, Gibbs CP, et al. Aneurysmal bone cyst. Am J Clin Oncol 2006;29:311.
100. Azouz EM, Saigal G, Rodriguez MM, et al. Langerhans' cell histiocytosis: pathology, imaging and treatment of skeletal involvement. Pediatr Radiol 2005;35:103.
101. Ghanem I. The management of osteoid osteoma: updates and controversies. Curr Opin Pediatr 2006;18:36.
102. Golant A, Lou JE, Erol B, et al. Pediatric osteoblastoma of the sternum: a new surgical technique for reconstruction after removal: case report and review of the literature. J Pediatr Orthop 2004;24:319.
103. Briccoli A, Malaguti C, Iannetti C, et al. Giant cell tumor of the rib. Skeletal Radiol 2003;32:107.
104. Widhe B, Bauer HC. Surgical treatment is decisive for outcome in chondrosarcoma of the chest wall: a population-based Scandinavian Sarcoma Group study of 106 patients. J Thorac Cardiovasc Surg 2009;137:610.
105. Riedel RF, Larrier N, Dodd L, et al. The clinical management of chondrosarcoma. Curr Treat Options Oncol 2009;10:94.
106. Burt M, Fulton M, Wessner-Dunlap S, et al. Primary bony and cartilaginous sarcomas of chest wall: results of therapy. Ann Thorac Surg 1992;54:226.
107. Deitch J, Crawford AH, Choudhury S. Osteogenic sarcoma of the rib: a case presentation and literature review. Spine (Phila Pa 1976) 2003;28:E74.
108. Carvajal R, Meyers P. Ewing's sarcoma and primitive neuroectodermal family of tumors. Hematol Oncol Clin North Am 2005;19:501.
109. Winer-Muram HT, Kauffman WM, Gronemeyer SA, et al. Primitive neuroectodermal tumors of the chest wall (Askin tumors): CT and MR findings. AJR Am J Roentgenol 1993;161:265.
110. Moser RP Jr, Davis MJ, Gilkey FW, et al. Primary Ewing sarcoma of rib. Radiographics 1990;10:899.
111. Shamberger RC, Laquaglia MP, Krailo MD, et al. Ewing sarcoma of the rib: results of an intergroup study with analysis of outcome by timing of resection. J Thorac Cardiovasc Surg 2000;119:1154.
112. Shamberger RC, LaQuaglia MP, Gebhardt MC, et al. Ewing sarcoma/primitive neuroectodermal tumor of the chest wall: impact of initial versus delayed resection on tumor margins, survival, and use of radiation therapy. Ann Surg 2003;238:563.
113. Schuck A, Hofmann J, Rube C, et al. Radiotherapy in Ewing's sarcoma and PNET of the chest wall: results of the trials CESS 81, CESS 86 and EICESS 92. Int J Radiat Oncol Biol Phys 1998;42:1001.
114. Skoracki RJ, Chang DW. Reconstruction of the chestwall and thorax. J Surg Oncol 2006;94:455.

Surgical and Nonresectional Therapies for Pulmonary Metastasis

Yifan Zheng, BS, Hiran C. Fernando, FRCS, MBBS*

KEYWORDS

- Pulmonary metastasis • Nonresectional therapy
- Video-assisted thoracic surgery • Surgical resection
- RFA • SBRT

Metastatic disease is a leading cause of cancer mortality, and the lungs are a common site of metastatic seeding. Tumors that exhibit preferential spread to the lungs include osteosarcoma, colon cancer, breast cancer, melanoma, and head and neck cancers. The lung is a prime metastatic target organ because of its anatomic and functional structure. It is highly vascular and rich in oxygen, providing pathways not just for metastatic seeding but also for a nutrient-rich environment for neoplastic growth.[1]

The standard treatment for isolated pulmonary metastasis has been surgical resection. The largest study performed to date on patients undergoing pulmonary metastasectomy reported better long-term outcomes in patients managed surgically in comparison with previously reported outcomes for patients managed nonsurgically.[2] This study, undertaken by the International Registry of Lung Metastases, accrued 5206 cases and found that the overall 5-year survival after resection ranged between 20% and 40%. According to the results, the significant prognostic factors of survival in patients undergoing pulmonary metastasectomy were the disease-free interval (DFI) from the primary tumor to the presentation of metastases, the tumor histology, and the number of metastases present. Patients with complete resections (as determined by preoperative radiological assessment, intraoperative findings, and postoperative pathologic analysis), a DFI of 36 months or more, a single metastatic nodule, and germ cell histology had the best observed prognosis.

While the treatment for pulmonary metastasis has historically been resection, newer therapies that do not require pulmonary resection have surfaced. Stereotactic body

Department of Cardiothoracic Surgery, Boston Medical Center, Boston University School of Medicine, 88 East Newton Street, Robinson B-402, Boston, MA 02118-2393, USA
* Corresponding author.
E-mail address: hiran.fernando@bmc.org

Surg Clin N Am 90 (2010) 1041–1051
doi:10.1016/j.suc.2010.06.003
0039-6109/10/$ – see front matter © 2010 Published by Elsevier Inc.

surgical.theclinics.com

radiation therapy (SBRT) and radiofrequency ablation (RFA) are 2 approaches that have been increasingly reported for pulmonary tumors.[3,4] Although these new therapies have yet to match the long-term success rates of surgical therapy, the techniques demonstrate good results in treating high-risk surgical candidates with metastatic lesions to the lungs that would otherwise be considered amenable to resection. Both have demonstrated 1-year survival post treatment of approximately 85%,[3,4] and 3-year survival rates of 46% for RFA patients and 25% for SBRT patients.[3,5] When compared with metastasectomy, which has 3-year survival rates as high as 78%[6] and long-term 10-year survival of 26%,[2] these methods are currently better reserved for the high-risk surgical patient. In this review, the management strategy for patients with metastatic pulmonary lesions will be discussed.

RESECTION OF PULMONARY METASTASES
Criteria for Surgical Resection

In 1947, Alexander and Haight described a series of pulmonary metastasectomies that led to the establishment of criteria for surgical resection.[7] These general criteria have evolved and can be summarized as follows:

1. The patient must be capable of tolerating the surgical procedure.
2. The patient's pulmonary function tests are supportive of the patient's ability to tolerate the loss of lung capacity resulting from the procedure.
3. The primary tumor has been controlled or is controllable, possibly by surgical means.
4. Any extrapulmonary disease is controlled or controllable, possibly by surgical means.

There have been several studies that have reported the outcomes of pulmonary metastasectomy. The overall operative mortality in the International Registry of Lung Metastases study was 1.3% and the median survival of patients with complete resections of tumor was 35 months.[2] The prognostic factors determined by this study have been supported by several other studies, which have also demonstrated 5-year survivals within the range listed by the Registry.[8,9] One particular report by Girard and colleagues[10] of 456 adult patients corroborated that the completeness of resection is prognostically significant to survival. These results indicate that metastasectomy is safe and can extend patient survival.

Given the strict indications before considering resection of metastases, nearly a third of patients with cancer will die with evidence of pulmonary metastasis found on autopsy.[11] The reason for this is in part because the patients who satisfy the criteria for resection are a smaller subgroup of those with pulmonary metastasis. One criterion that often disqualifies a patient from metastasectomy is the lack of controllable extrapulmonary disease. Some tumor types are more likely to metastasize to a single site, such as the lungs, whereas others have a more pervasive spread. Sarcomas, renal cell cancers, and head and neck cancers are examples of cancers with preferential spread to the lungs, whereas breast, melanoma, and colorectal cancers often spread to multiple sites throughout the body so many of these patients will not be candidates for pulmonary resection.[8] For patients that can be treated with resection there are 2 main approaches: open resection or a minimally invasive approach using video-assisted thoracic surgery (VATS).

Surgical Approaches

Once the decision has been made to perform a metastasectomy, the approach taken is dependent on the extent and location of the tumor. Disease that has spread to both lungs will usually be treated by an open approach. A median sternotomy, for example, provides bilateral exposure but is limited by poor access to the posterior lung regions, particularly the left lower lobe. The clamshell incision, when compared with the median sternotomy, provides better bilateral exposure but requires the sacrifice of both of the internal thoracic arteries. The median sternotomy and clamshell incision have their limitations, but both are less painful than a standard posterolateral thoracotomy. However, a posterolateral thoracotomy provides excellent exposure of the entire lung and is the preferred open approach for disease limited to one lung.[7]

The least painful surgical approach for metastasectomy is VATS. In a study using questionnaires involving 165 thoracotomy patients and 178 VATS patients, less pain and shoulder dysfunction was reported in the VATS group in the early (<1 year) post-operative period.[12] In a study comparing VATS with open segmentectomy for stage I non–small cell lung cancer, VATS patients had a significantly shorter ($P<.001$) median hospital stay of 5 days whereas the open segmentectomy patients had a median stay of 7 days.[13] The same study also showed that 15.4% of the VATS patients had pulmonary complications compared with 29.8% of the thoracotomy group ($P = .012$). A study by Ninomiya and colleagues[14] also noted less pulmonary compromise in patients after VATS when compared with open metastasectomy patients. The VATS group had an early and late decrease in vital capacity of 16.2% and 2%, respectively, which were both significantly less than the early and late post-thoracotomy vital capacity reductions, which were 33% and 17.8%, respectively. These studies support the argument that VATS may be a less morbid approach than thoracotomy.

Despite this, there are concerns that with a VATS approach, palpation of the lung will be limited and metastatic disease will be missed. This concern was supported by a study done at Memorial Sloan-Kettering Cancer Center.[15] In this prospective study, following VATS resection an immediate thoracotomy was performed to confirm resection of all palpable metastases. The study was closed prematurely because of significant results in the first 15 patients enrolled. At thoracotomy, 10 of 15 patients had additional malignant nodules that were not identified on their computed tomography (CT) scans or during their VATS procedures.

However, in 2002 a European study compared pulmonary metastasis patients treated with VATS alone with patients treated with VATS followed by a thoracotomy.[16] There were significantly ($P = .049$) more complications in the thoracotomy group, and 2-year overall survivals were similar for both groups (67% and 70%), suggesting that VATS may be a reasonable approach.[16] One reason for a difference in these conclusions may be that the second study was limited to patients with an isolated metastasis whereas the earlier Memorial Sloan-Kettering study allowed 1 to 2 ipsilateral tumors. The Memorial Sloan-Kettering study was performed in the earlier days of VATS and before the availability of newer generation helical CT scanners that may be more sensitive in detecting small metastatic pulmonary lesions.[17] Furthermore, an unknown factor to consider is the significance of leaving behind disease that is occult on radiological imaging. In most studies of metastasectomy, survival is better in patients who have complete resection than in those with incomplete resection, but patients with incomplete resection have known gross disease that is left behind. The issue of occult disease was addressed in a study comparing metastasectomy for sarcoma via a sternotomy (which allowed bimanual palpation of both lungs) or a thoracotomy (which allowed palpation of just one lung) approach.[18] Although sternotomy detected unsuspected bilateral disease, there was no difference in survival between the 2 groups.

A technique that has been suggested to help identify lesions that may be missed by standard radiographic imaging is hand-assisted thoracoscopic surgery (HATS). HATS involves the introduction of a hand port during a VATS procedure. In a HATS study conducted by Detterbeck and Egan,[19] 5 of 16 patients had additional nodules identified that were not seen on preoperative CT scan. However, in only 3 of these 5 patients were these nodules malignant.

Based on this ongoing discussion, it is appropriate to conclude that VATS is a reasonable initial approach for patients with limited disease (1–2 metastases) in the outer third of the lung. For patients with more extensive disease, where the chance of additional metastases is higher, thoracotomy is preferred. In addition, for those with more deeply situated disease, thoracotomy is preferred because it will be easier to tailor the resection to optimize sparing of lung parenchyma, but still remove the metastases with an acceptable margin.

NONRESECTIONAL LOCAL THERAPY FOR PULMONARY METASTASES

Two forms of local ablative therapies have been introduced to treat pulmonary tumors, namely RFA and SBRT. Although for non–small cell lung cancer there is probably more reported experience with SBRT than with RFA, the converse is true for pulmonary metastases. With both therapies, the studies are relatively small with limited follow-up, making direct comparison with surgical resection limited. Despite this the early data are encouraging, as is now discussed.

Radiofrequency Ablation

RFA was originally described for the treatment of hepatic tumors, but there is an increasing number of reports in the literature of its use for pulmonary malignancies.[20–22] RFA consists of an alternating current that oscillates between active and dispersive electrodes. The active electrode is placed within the tumor usually with CT guidance, and the dispersive electrode—usually an electrosurgical return pad—is placed on the patient. The generator provides the current that passes between these electrodes. The ions in the tissue oscillate to follow the direction of the alternating current, resulting in the frictional heating of the tissue. A region of necrosis is generated by this frictional heating of the tumor tissue around the active electrode. For normal cells, temperatures greater than 60°C are required to cause cell death. However, cancer cells are more sensitive to heat, and temperatures as low as 41°C can induce cell death.[23] To date the Food and Drug Administration of the United States has approved 3 RFA systems for use in soft tissue. Although there is no specific lung indication, percutaneous ablations of lung tumors are commonly performed, and Medicare has assigned the procedure a specific code (32998). The 3 commercially available RFA systems in the United States are the Boston Scientific (Natick, MA, USA) system (BOS), RITA Medical (Manchester, GA, USA) system (RITA), and the Valleylab (Boulder, CO, USA) system (VL).[21] Although all systems cause local heating in and immediately adjacent to the tumor, each system has a different design. The active electrode of the VL system consists of either a cluster of 3 parallel needles or just a single needle with tips that are infused with cold water. The water infusion cools the electrode to prevent charring of the tissue immediately around the active probe. The active electrodes of the BOS and RITA systems consist of multiple expandable tines. The RITA system can also disperse saline into the tissue during ablation, which is believed to increase the thermal lesion by promoting conduction through the dispersed saline. The VL and BOS systems are impedance-based systems, meaning that the end point of ablation occurs when impedance in the tissue rises significantly, preventing further current flow and local heating. The RITA system uses temperature and time to determine the end point of ablation.

As mentioned, RFA has been used successfully for the treatment of hepatic tumors. In the liver, RFA has provided necrosis rates of 70% to 98%.[22] In the lung, RFA has been shown to be effective for Stage I and II primary non–small cell lung cancer, with better results for smaller tumors.[24] In an early report of RFA, one patient developed massive hemoptysis almost 3 weeks after ablation of a central lung tumor.[24] For this reason, the authors believe that RFA should be reserved for treating tumors that are not directly abutting or close to mediastinal blood vessels. In general, the indications for RFA are similar to that for resection of metastases, although this procedure has been reserved for a higher operative risk group. In summary, a patient qualifies for RFA if the following criteria are fulfilled[25,26]:

1. The patient is determined to be an unsuitable candidate for surgery.
2. All tumor lesions are small in diameter.
3. Tumor lesions are not abutting mediastinal structures.
4. The primary tumor has been controlled or is controllable.
5. There is a limited number of metastatic nodules.

An important difference between RFA and resection is that the treatment margin will be unknown because no tissue is sent for pathologic analysis.[25] The goal in RFA is to achieve 100% ablation with an ablation zone that is ideally 1 cm larger than the original lesion,[25] but this has proved to be a challenge. In an RFA study of pulmonary metastases, ablation was performed at thoracotomy before an immediate wedge resection, providing histologic analysis of the ablated lesion.[27] This study found that 100% ablation was obtained in only 39% of the study population, although 89% of the patients had 90% or greater ablation of their metastasis. The investigators commented that there was a possibility of the remaining viable tumor cells dying off a few days after the procedure, indicating that early pathologic analysis may underestimate the effectiveness of tumor ablation.

One of the difficulties in evaluating the literature relating to RFA (and even for metastases in general) is that most series include several different tumor types. Perhaps the most experience with single-histology metastases has been with colorectal carcinoma. In one prospective study of 55 patients with colorectal metastases to the lungs, the 1-year survival after RFA was 85% and the 3-year survival was 46%.[3] An earlier study done by the same group found that at 1-year follow-up, more than 60% of the treated metastatic nodules remained undetectable, had decreased in size, or were stable.[28] Although these rates are not as promising as the best 5-year survival rates of 40% as mentioned for metastasectomy, they do reflect the promise and efficacy of RFA as a resection alternative for surgically unsuitable patients.

More recently, 2 new studies published in 2009 report the outcomes of ablation for patients with pulmonary metastases with different histologies. In one report, 39 patients with inoperable renal cell metastases underwent RFA. Patients were divided into 2 groups. The first group, with 6 or fewer nodules with none measuring greater than 6 cm, was treated with curative intent. The second group, with more than 6 nodules or with nodules larger than 6 cm, was treated with palliative intent. Of note, in the group treated with curative intent 1-year, 3-year, and 5-year overall survivals were 100%. Recurrence-free survivals were lower, 1-year, 3-year, and 5-year rates being 92%, 23%, and 23%, respectively.[29] Another study involving 22 patients with metastases of various histologies demonstrated a 2-year and median survival of 68% and 29 months, respectively.[30] Lesion size was again found to be a prognostic factor for both survival and recurrence.

In terms of the morbidity and mortality associated with RFA, an international survey found the procedure to have little of either.[31] A total of 493 RFA procedures were performed across 7 centers and of that only 2 deaths were reported (0.4%). Complications occurred in no more than 30% of the nearly 500 cases. Pneumothorax was the most common complication associated with ablative procedures. In terms of complication severity, pneumothorax can be regarded as relatively benign. The Common Toxicity Criteria used in oncology trials only regards pneumothorax as a grade 3 event if sclerosis or surgery is required. In addition, a chest tube is always required after resection, but not always after RFA. This study demonstrates that RFA is a safe alternative that can be effective for treating pulmonary metastases in the high operative risk patient.

Stereotactic Body Radiation Therapy

SBRT allows for the delivery of high doses of radiation, which have been found to have better local tumor control.[32] Because of the high doses normally used in SBRT, the number of fractions are usually fewer and the biologically equivalent dose (BED) is much higher than with conventional radiation techniques.

SBRT has been successfully applied to benign and malignant conditions of the brain and spine since its conception in the 1950s.[33] It is only in the last decade that SBRT has become more commonly used for lung tumors. In the past this was difficult to achieve because of respiratory motion and the proximity of vital structures limiting traditional radiation plans.

Respiratory displacements are greatest near the diaphragm and least near the apices and the carina. One method of minimizing the effects of respiratory motion is by breath holding, which is often used in combination with an abdominal compression device to limit the caudal movement of the diaphragm. Another method used to compensate for respiratory motion is respiratory gating. A CT scanner takes serial images so as to define the exact position of the tumor as it relates to the specific breathing pattern of the patient, and the radiation dose is administered during the phase of the breathing cycle that maximizes tumor exposure and minimizes surrounding tissue exposure. Lastly, a technique known as dynamic tracking can also be used to minimize the effects of respiratory motion. In this technique, gold fiducials are percutaneously implanted next to the tumor, allowing the SBRT linear accelerator system to localize the tumor in space. This goal is accomplished by recording the breathing movements of the patient and combining that information with

Table 1
Survival after treatment for colorectal metastasis

Study	N	Median Follow-Up (months)	Median Survival (months)	Survival Rates at:		
				2 Years	3 Years	5 Years
Open[35]	144	N/A	42[b]	N/A	N/A	44%
Open[36]	153	35	39	64%	N/A	37%
VATS[37]	80	N/A	35[b]	N/A	48.4%	30.8%
VATS[38a]	24	29	32[b]	N/A	N/A	49.5%
RFA[3]	55	24	33	64%	46%	N/A
RFA[39]	18	27.5	N/A	78%	57%	57%
SBRT[40]	13	28	N/A	75.5%	64.7%	N/A

Abbreviations: N/A, not available; RFA, radiofrequency ablation; SBRT, stereotactic body radiation therapy; VATS, video-assisted thoracic surgery.
  [a] Single metastasis.
  [b] Median survival not reported in text but estimated from survival curve in manuscript.

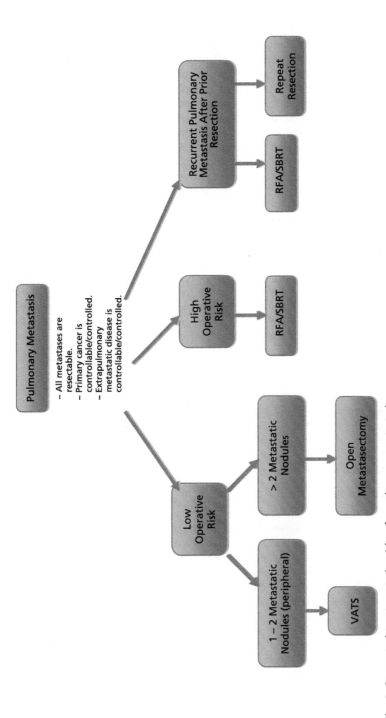

Fig. 1. Suggested treatment algorithm for pulmonary metastasis.

sequential radiographs of the fiducials so that radiation can be delivered during the respiratory cycle. This technique has the added advantage of shorter treatment times than breath holding.

The patients who qualify for this ablative therapy fulfill criteria very similar to those of RFA. However, one advantage of SBRT as compared with RFA is that it is possible to treat tumors close to the mediastinum,[26] although the radiation dose will need to be reduced to minimize toxicity. At present there are limited data on the use of SBRT specifically for pulmonary metastases. One study of SBRT for pulmonary metastases reported that in 30 patients treated with curative intent the 1-, 2-, and 3-year overall survivals were 71%, 38%, and 25%, respectively.[5] It should be noted that most patients in this series had undergone other therapies for their metastatic disease, and the median time from the first presentation of their metastatic disease to referral for SBRT was 14.8 months. Another study done of SBRT included 13 patients with solitary lung metastases.[4] Patients were treated with a total of 60 Gy delivered in 3 fractions. The 1-year survival for this group of patients was 62%.

A multi-institutional phase 1/2 trial of SBRT for pulmonary metastases was recently reported.[34] Among the 38 patients, a total of 63 metastatic lesions were treated. Local control (of the treated lesions) was 100% and 96% at 1 and 2 years, and median survival was 19 months. These studies demonstrate that SBRT is feasible for patients with pulmonary metastases. One consideration, however, is that it may be challenging to treat several lesions and avoid morbidity such as pneumonitis from radiation toxicity, particularly in the high-risk patient. On the other hand, it is now feasible to use a combination of approaches (resection, ablation, and SBRT) and tailor the approach for a particular patient depending on factors such as number of lesions, lesion location, pulmonary function, and operative risk.

SUMMARY

Metastasectomy has been well established as a reasonable approach for patients with pulmonary oligometastases. RFA and SBRT are also effective therapies that may be a less morbid approach for these patients, who may develop further metastases even after complete resection is undertaken. However, because we cannot be certain that all targeted metastatic lung nodules will be obliterated by either SBRT or RFA, these alternative approaches should be reserved for patients at high operative risk. At present, no comparative studies of these modalities have been undertaken, and interpreting the data that are available is difficult because of the multiple tumor types reported in metastases series. Perhaps the best single-histology data that are available concern colorectal cancer metastases. **Table 1** provides a summary of outcomes for colorectal metastases treated with resection, RFA, and SBRT. On initial review, it would appear that survival may be as good or even better than surgery. However, the RFA and SBRT series are limited by smaller sample sizes and shorter follow-up. These data are nevertheless intriguing, and a future randomized trial is not unreasonable.

Until further data are available, resection should be the approach of choice. **Fig. 1** outlines a suggested algorithm when approaching the patient with pulmonary metastases. Although not discussed in detail, RFA or SBRT may be reasonable for patients presenting with recurrent metastatic disease after previous resection, even in patients with good pulmonary function. Reoperation will be more challenging, with a higher possibility of complications such as bleeding or prolonged air leak, and it is even more likely that such patients will present with further disease after resection. Also, having potentially lost lung function due to resection in the prior metastasectomy, ablation may minimize any additional loss. As further data become available (ideally from a randomized trial), it is likely that this algorithm will be further modified.

REFERENCES

1. Krishnan K, Khanna C, Helman LJ. The molecular biology of pulmonary metastasis. Thorac Surg Clin 2006;16(2):115–24.
2. Long-term results of lung metastasectomy: prognostic analyses based on 5206 cases. The International Registry of Lung Metastases. J Thorac Cardiovasc Surg 1997;113(1):37–49.
3. Yan TD, King J, Sjarif A, et al. Percutaneous radiofrequency ablation of pulmonary metastases from colorectal carcinoma: prognostic determinants for survival. Ann Surg Oncol 2006;13(11):1529–37.
4. Coon D, Gokhale AS, Burton SA, et al. Fractionated stereotactic body radiation therapy in the treatment of primary, recurrent, and metastatic lung tumors: the role of positron emission tomography/computed tomography-based treatment planning. Clin Lung Cancer 2008;9(4):217–21.
5. Okunieff P, Petersen AL, Philip A, et al. Stereotactic body radiation therapy (SBRT) for lung metastases. Acta Oncol 2006;45(7):808–17.
6. Onaitis MW, Petersen RP, Haney JC, et al. Prognostic factors for recurrence after pulmonary resection of colorectal cancer metastases. Ann Thorac Surg 2009;87(6):1684–8.
7. Davidson RS, Nwogu CE, Brentjens MJ, et al. The surgical management of pulmonary metastasis: current concepts. Surg Oncol 2001;10(1–2):35–42.
8. Abecasis N, Cortez F, Bettencourt A, et al. Surgical treatment of lung metastases: prognostic factors for long-term survival. J Surg Oncol 1999;72(4):193–8.
9. Koodziejski L, Góralczyk J, Dyczek S, et al. The role of surgery in lung metastases. Eur J Surg Oncol 1999;25(4):410–7.
10. Girard P, Baldeyrou P, Le Chevalier T, et al. Surgical resection of pulmonary metastases. Up to what number? Am J Respir Crit Care Med 1994;149(2 Pt 1): 469–76.
11. Ollila DW, Morton DL. Surgical resection as the treatment of choice for melanoma metastatic to the lung. Chest Surg Clin N Am 1998;8(1):183–96.
12. Landreneau RJ, Mack MJ, Hazelrigg SR, et al. Prevalence of chronic pain after pulmonary resection by thoracotomy or video-assisted thoracic surgery. J Thorac Cardiovasc Surg 1994;107(4):1079–85 [discussion: 1085–6].
13. Schuchert MJ, Pettiford BL, Pennathur A, et al. Anatomic segmentectomy for stage I non-small-cell lung cancer: comparison of video-assisted thoracic surgery versus open approach. J Thorac Cardiovasc Surg 2009;138(6): 1318–25. e1.
14. Ninomiya M, Nakajima J, Tanaka M, et al. Effects of lung metastasectomy on respiratory function. Jpn J Thorac Cardiovasc Surg 2001;49(1):17–20.
15. McCormack PM, Bains MS, Begg CB, et al. Role of video-assisted thoracic surgery in the treatment of pulmonary metastases: results of a prospective trial. Ann Thorac Surg 1996;62(1):213–6 [discussion: 216–7].
16. Mutsaerts EL, Zoetmulder FA, Meijer S, et al. Long term survival of thoracoscopic metastasectomy vs metastasectomy by thoracotomy in patients with a solitary pulmonary lesion. Eur J Surg Oncol 2002;28(8):864–8.
17. Margaritora S, Porziella V, D'Andrilli A, et al. Pulmonary metastases: can accurate radiological evaluation avoid thoracotomic approach? Eur J Cardiothorac Surg 2002;21(6):1111–4.

18. Roth JA, Pass HI, Wesley MN, et al. Comparison of median sternotomy and thoracotomy for resection of pulmonary metastases in patients with adult soft-tissue sarcomas. Ann Thorac Surg 1986;42(2):134–8.

19. Detterbeck FC, Egan TM. Thoracoscopy using a substernal handport for palpation. Ann Thorac Surg 2004;78(3):1031–6.

20. Curley SA, Izzo F, Delrio P, et al. Radiofrequency ablation of unresectable primary and metastatic hepatic malignancies: results in 123 patients. Ann Surg 1999;230(1):1–8.

21. Fernando HC. Radiofrequency ablation to treat non-small cell lung cancer and pulmonary metastases. Ann Thorac Surg 2008;85(2):S780–4.

22. Curley SA, Izzo F. Laparoscopic radiofrequency. Ann Surg Oncol 2000;7(2):78–9.

23. Giovanella BC, Lohman WA, Heidelberger C. Effects of elevated temperatures and drugs on the viability of L1210 leukemia cells. Cancer Res 1970;30(6): 1623–31.

24. Herrera LJ, Fernando HC, Perry Y, et al. Radiofrequency ablation of pulmonary malignant tumors in nonsurgical candidates. J Thorac Cardiovasc Surg 2003; 125(4):929–37.

25. Ketchedjian A, Daly B, Luketich J, et al. Minimally invasive techniques for managing pulmonary metastases: video-assisted thoracic surgery and radiofrequency ablation. Thorac Surg Clin 2006;16(2):157–65.

26. Fernando HC, Ghulam A. "Alternatives to surgical resection for non-small lung cancer." Pearson's thoracic and esophageal surgery. 3rd edition. Philadelphia: Churchill and Livingston; 2008. p. 796–803.

27. Schneider T, Warth A, Herpel E, et al. Intraoperative radiofrequency ablation of lung metastases and histologic evaluation. Ann Thorac Surg 2009;87(2):379–84.

28. Steinke K, Glenn D, King J, et al. Percutaneous imaging-guided radiofrequency ablation in patients with colorectal pulmonary metastases: 1-year follow-up. Ann Surg Oncol 2004;11(2):207–12.

29. Soga N, Yamakado K, Gohara H, et al. Percutaneous radiofrequency ablation for unresectable pulmonary metastases from renal cell carcinoma. BJU Int 2009;104(6):790–4.

30. Pennathur A, Abbas G, Qureshi I, et al. Radiofrequency ablation for the treatment of pulmonary metastases. Ann Thorac Surg 2009;87(4):1030–6 [discussion: 1036–9].

31. Steinke K, Sewell PE, Dupuy D, et al. Pulmonary radiofrequency ablation—an international study survey. Anticancer Res 2004;24(1):339–43.

32. Baumann M, Appold S, Petersen C, et al. Dose and fractionation concepts in the primary radiotherapy of non-small cell lung cancer. Lung Cancer 2001;33 (Suppl 1):S35–45.

33. Cesaretti JA, Pennathur A, Rosenstein BS, et al. Stereotactic radiosurgery for thoracic malignancies. Ann Thorac Surg 2008;85(2):S785–91.

34. Rusthoven KE, Kavanagh BD, Burri SH, et al. Multi-institutional phase I/II trial of stereotactic body radiation therapy for lung metastases. J Clin Oncol 2009; 27(10):1579–84.

35. McCormack PM, Burt ME, Bains MS, et al. Lung resection for colorectal metastases. 10-year results. Arch Surg 1992;127(12):1403–6.

36. Yedibela S, Klein P, Feuchter K, et al. Surgical management of pulmonary metastases from colorectal cancer in 153 patients. Ann Surg Oncol 2006;13(11): 1538–44.

37. Landreneau RJ, De Giacomo T, Mack MJ, et al. Therapeutic video-assisted thoracoscopic surgical resection of colorectal pulmonary metastases. Eur J Cardiothorac Surg 2000;18(6):671–6 [discussion: 676–7].

38. DiGiacomo T, Rendina EA, Venuta F, et al. Thoracoscopic resection of solitary lung metastases from colorectal cancer is a viable therapeutic option. Chest 1999;115(5):1441–3.
39. Simon CJ, Dupuy DE, DiPetrillo TA, et al. Pulmonary radiofrequency ablation: long-term safety and efficacy in 153 patients. Radiology 2007;243(1):268–75.
40. Kim MS, Yoo SY, Cho CK, et al. Stereotactic body radiation therapy using three fractions for isolated lung recurrence from colorectal cancer. Oncology 2009;76(3):212–9.

Endoscopic Evaluation of the Tracheobronchial Tree and Mediastinal Lymph Nodes

Daniel P. Raymond, MD, Thomas J. Watson, MD*

KEYWORDS

- Endoscopic evaluation • Bronchoscopy
- Endobronchial ultrasound • Mediastinal lymph nodes

Although attempts to cannulate the upper aerodigestive tract date back to the days of Hippocrates, the origins of modern bronchoscopy begin in the eighteenth century with the development of instruments to illuminate cavities of the human body, such as the Lichtleiter developed by Philipp Bozzini (1773–1809).[1] Antonio Jean Desormeaux (1815–1894) a French urologist, coined the term *endoscopy* and is often considered the Father of Endoscopy because of his development of a urethroscope illuminated by a chemical reagent. Subsequently, Adolf Kussmaul (1822–1902) performed the first direct esophagoscopy in 1868 using mirrors and a gasoline lamp on a sword swallower, and Johann von Mikulicz (1850–1905) introduced the first electrically illuminated esophagoscope. Laryngologists Gustav Killian (1860–1921) and Alfred Kirstein (1863–1922) later championed the assessment of the airways using a modified endoscope and the modern era of bronchoscopy was born. Subsequent innovations, including the distal illuminating endoscope (Chevalier Jackson), the fiberoptic light source (Edwin Broyles), and the flexible fiberoptic bronchoscope (Shigeto Ikeda), have resulted in a revolution in technology and technique that has altered the face of modern medicine.[1]

RIGID BRONCHOSCOPY

Rigid bronchoscopy is not only of historical interest but remains an essential tool for evaluation and management of the airway. Although the indications for its use have decreased considerably with advancements in flexible technology, rigid

Division of Thoracic and Foregut Surgery, Department of Surgery, University of Rochester School of Medicine and Dentistry, 601 Elmwood Avenue, Box Surgery, Rochester, NY 14642, USA
* Corresponding author.
E-mail address: Thomas_watson@urmc.rochester.edu

Surg Clin N Am 90 (2010) 1053–1063
doi:10.1016/j.suc.2010.06.007
0039-6109/10/$ – see front matter © 2010 Elsevier Inc. All rights reserved.

bronchoscopy is indispensable for the evaluation of obstructing airway lesions and is a useful therapeutic instrument; its large diameter facilitates removal of airway foreign bodies, clearance of blood clots or thick secretions, debridement and extraction of airway neoplasms, and dilation of benign or malignant stenoses of the major airways.

Rigid bronchoscopy is generally performed under general anesthesia, using a port on the side of the scope to provide ventilation (**Fig. 1**). Air/gas flow is through the distal tip of the scope as well as through side holes near the tip. For situations where the scope will be positioned proximally for an extended period of time (eg, obstructing proximal tracheal tumors or benign stenoses), the side holes may need to be occluded with metal tape to prevent leakage of air/gas into the pharynx. Preprocedural knowledge of the etiology and location of the underlying airway pathology and patients' pulmonary reserve is critical, and generally obtained from the history, physical examination findings, and preoperative chest radiographs including CT. Such information can help to plan interventions and anticipate potential pitfalls or complications. Proper ventilation and administration of anesthetic agents is essential and management plans should be thoroughly discussed with the anesthesia team before induction.

Patients are often first intubated in a standard manner using an endotracheal tube. Once patients have been adequately induced and positioned, the tube is exchanged for the rigid bronchoscope. The mouth is then packed to control air leaks and to maintain positive pressure ventilation while the anesthesiologist continuously monitors the adequacy of gas exchange. The bronchoscopist must be careful to visualize the vocal cords to avoid injury during scope insertion, turning the scope so that its wider diameter is oriented in the anteroposterior plane to facilitate passage. Patients' teeth should be protected with a mouth guard or finger while the scope is being manipulated. The tendency to lever the rigid scope against patients' upper teeth must be avoided to prevent injury.

An important decision when preparing to intervene in patients with a near obstructing tracheal lesion is whether to try to keep patients spontaneously breathing or induce paralysis. Although keeping patients spontaneously breathing adds an element of safety if intubating the airway is difficult or an equipment malfunction occurs, it requires a skilled anesthesiologist to balance adequate sedation and continued spontaneous ventilation in patients with critical airway obstruction.[2] Further, coughing or an unexpected movement by patients may precipitate bleeding or injury that can complicate an already complex situation. These issues are negated by inducing paralysis upon initiation of the procedure, but the bronchoscopist must be experienced and skilled at intubating the airway with the rigid bronchoscope and rapidly obtaining a satisfactory airway because ventilation by mask is unlikely to be an option. This factor is particularly true for proximal airway lesions, typically tight benign strictures.

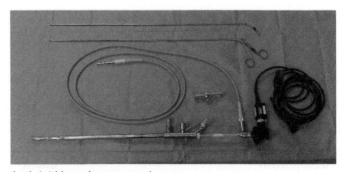

Fig. 1. Standard rigid bronchoscopy equipment.

In distal lesions ventilation through the rigid scope above the lesion, or with a jet ventilator, may be possible at least for a short period of time until an adequate airway is established by either balloon dilating the lesion, dilating or coring it out with the rigid bronchoscope, or destroying the obstructing tissue with argon beam coagulation, laser, or cryotherapy. Prior to the start of procedure it is critical to ensure that all necessary equipment is available and fully functional, as little time may be afforded to establish an airway, particularly in debilitated patients with poor cardiopulmonary reserve. Minor mistakes in preparedness and judgment can result in catastrophic outcomes in these commonly tenuous, life or death scenarios (**Figs. 2–4**).

Limitations of rigid bronchoscopy include the need for general anesthesia; potential difficulty in passing the scope because of anatomic problems, such as kyphosis or difficulty visualizing the larynx; the risk for dental injury; inability to visualize upper lobe and distal airway pathology; and the risk for airway injury. The morbidity of rigid bronchoscopy is generally considered to be higher than that of flexible bronchoscopy,[3] although patient selection remains a significant confounding factor and in certain clinical situations the rigid instrument is absolutely essential.

FLEXIBLE BRONCHOSCOPY

Since the introduction of the first fiberoptic flexible video bronchoscope in the late 1980s, a revolution in technology has resulted in the widespread dissemination of flexible instruments worldwide. Flexible bronchoscopy is now considered a basic tool for the visualization and biopsy of the tracheobronchial tree and is used by numerous specialties. Advantages relative to rigid bronchoscopy include the ability to perform the procedure with local or intravenous (IV) sedation in an outpatient setting, superior optics and video capabilities, the ability to assess smaller and more distal airways, the relative ease of passage and use, patient tolerance with a low rate of complications, and a quick learning curve.

Flexible bronchoscopy is most commonly performed under IV sedation augmented by topical anesthesia. Anesthetic agents may be delivered to the pharynx, larynx, and trachea before the procedure via nebulizer, transtracheal injection, or under direct visualization, as well as during the procedure directly through the working channel of the bronchoscope. Toxicities related to application of topical anesthesia are a common cause of procedure-associated morbidity.[3] The maximum dose of topical

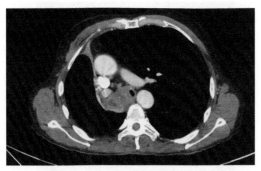

Fig. 2. High-grade carinal obstruction caused by large carinal squamous cell carcinoma in 59-year-old smoker presenting in respiratory distress. Patient was managed with emergent rigid bronchoscopy to establish adequate airway to the left side. Subsequent rigid bronchoscopic interventions reestablished patency of the right main stem bronchus permitting the patient to be discharged from the hospital to pursue additional treatments.

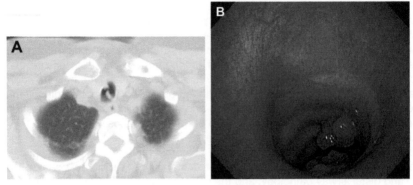

Fig. 3. (*A* and *B*) CT and bronchoscopic images of tracheal papillomas in a patient presenting with cough.

agents, therefore, should be determined before the procedure and strictly adhered to throughout. Intravenous sedation requires appropriate personnel and hemodynamic monitoring as well as supervised recovery. The safety of patients and health care personnel is of paramount importance. Safeguards include use of an appropriate

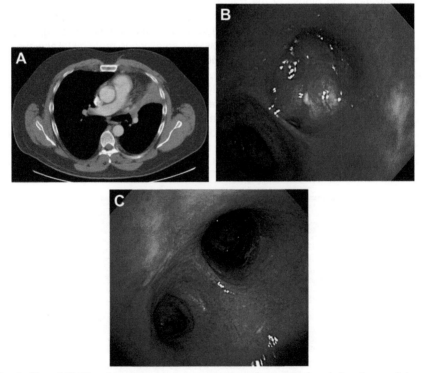

Fig. 4. (*A* and *B*) CT and bronchoscopic images of a left upper lobe obstructing endobronchial lesion in a patient presenting with dyspnea and a l abnormality. (*C*) Biopsy subsequently revealed endobronchial hamartomas, which were successfully removed by bronchoscopic techniques.

environment and attire by practitioners to prevent droplet transmission of an infectious agent.

The bronchoscopic equipment, including light source, video hardware and monitor, are often contained on a convenient portable cart that permits use in numerous settings. After adequate topical and IV sedation are achieved, the bronchoscope is inserted either through the transnasal or transoral route. A bite block is strongly recommended for the latter to prevent damage to the scope. The hypopharynx and vocal cords are initially inspected and additional topical anesthesia may be applied. Subsequently, the trachea is inspected and a systematic examination of the airways is undertaken. Photographs and video are useful for documentation of pathology. Based on the findings, various diagnostic procedures may be undertaken, including washings, bronchoalveolar lavage, brushings, and biopsy.

Adjuncts to Diagnostic Bronchoscopy

Bronchial washings are performed by instilling small amounts of normal saline through the working channel of the bronchoscope and then aspirating that fluid to obtain specimens for cytologic and microbiologic examination. Bronchoalveolar lavage (BAL) is a more specific technique for obtaining samples of cellular and noncellular contents of the distal airways and alveoli. The technique is generally performed by wedging the bronchoscope in a subsegmental bronchus in the region of clinical suspicion. An aliquot of saline (30–50 mL) is then instilled, aspirated, and the contents discarded to wash out contaminants from the proximal airways. Subsequently, several additional aliquots are instilled, suctioned, and collected in a sterile specimen trap for analysis. The total volume of retrieved fluid is variable and should be recorded as a measure of specimen adequacy. The lack of a standardized technique remains a challenge relative to the interpretation of results and comparisons between institutions. It is recommended that each center derive a standard technique based on professional society guidelines.[4]

Bronchial brushings and endobronchial biopsies may be obtained with the added guidance of fluoroscopy for peripheral lesions. Transbronchial needle biopsies may be undertaken using a blind technique or with ultrasound guidance. The diagnostic yield of bronchoscopy in comparison to other techniques for evaluation of pulmonary pathology is an issue commonly confronted by thoracic surgeons. The decision to pursue a bronchoscopic biopsy as opposed to evaluation of expectorated sputum, radiologically guided transthoracic needle biopsy, or surgical biopsy by video-assisted or open technique requires knowledge of the diagnostic yield of various procedures as well as the particulars of the presenting pathology and risk profile of patients. **Table 1** summarizes a meta-analysis performed by Schreiber and McCrory[5] evaluating the performance characteristics of sputum analysis, flexible bronchoscopy, and transthoracic needle biopsy (TTNB) in the evaluation of patients with suspected lung cancer. Factors, including lesion size and location, have significant impact on the sensitivity of all the studies. Not surprisingly, the sensitivity of bronchoscopy is highest for central lesions and lowest for small, peripheral lesions, with diagnostic yields reported as low as 14%[6] in the latter scenario. The diagnostic yield for peripheral lesions is superior for TTNB, although the risk profile for this procedure, including a pneumothorax rate of 10% to 54%,[7] must also be considered.

Recently, additional technologies have been added to the bronchoscopist's armamentarium to enhance the diagnostic yield. These technologies include endobronchial ultrasound (EBUS) and electromagnetic navigational bronchoscopy (ENB).

Table 1	
Sensitivities of bronchoscopic biopsy techniques	
Technique	**Pooled Sensitivity**
Sputum cytology	0.66
Central lesions	0.71
Peripheral lesions	0.49
Flexible bronchoscopy[a]	—
Central lesions	0.88
Peripheral lesions	0.69
Peripheral >2 cm	0.62
Peripheral <2 cm	0.33
Transthoracic needle biopsy	0.90
>1.5 cm	0.94
<1.5cm	0.78

[a] Utilizing standard techniques including biopsy, brushing, washing bronchoalveolar lavage, and transbronchial needle aspiration.
Data from Schreiber D, McCrory DC. Performance characteristics of different modalities for diagnosis of suspected lung cancer: summary of published evidence. Chest 2003;123(Suppl 1):115S–28S.

Endobronchial Ultrasound

Endobronchial ultrasound has permitted the real-time imaging of structures adjacent to the tracheobronchial tree, enhancing the diagnostic capabilities of the bronchoscopist, and is currently available in 2 forms: radial and linear arrays. The radial EBUS is a 20 MHz rotating transducer that is introduced through the working channel of a standard flexible bronchoscope. The tip of the catheter is fitted with a balloon that permits coupling with the bronchial wall. The radial ultrasound creates a 360° image perpendicular to the axis of the probe. Biopsy requires removal of the catheter and therefore cannot be done in real time. In contrast, the linear EBUS is the combination of a curved linear array ultrasound with a 35° forward-viewing bronchoscope. A specially designed biopsy needle is used with the scope to provide real-time imaging during biopsy (**Fig. 5**). The utility of the linear EBUS is, however, limited by its size and it is generally used for biopsying mediastinal and hilar lymph nodes or masses.

Before the introduction of EBUS, transbronchial needle biopsies (TBNB) were obtained in a blind fashion with needle placement based on radiographic evidence of lymph node pathology, the endoscopist's knowledge of mediastinal anatomy, and endobronchial evidence of adjacent pathology (eg, carinal widening, luminal compression, or mucosal irregularity). The sensitivity of this technique ranges from 34% to 78%, depending on the prevalence of benign mediastinal pathology in the patient population.[8] In a direct comparison of traditional TBNB with EBUS-TBNB, Wallace and colleagues[9] revealed a superior sensitivity of the EBUS technique in evaluating the mediastinal lymph nodes of subjects with suspected cancer (69% vs 36%; $P = .003$). The addition of endoscopic ultrasound examination and transesophageal biopsy further enhanced the diagnostic accuracy of the evaluation. Finally, a recent meta-analysis by Gu and colleagues[10] revealed a sensitivity of 93% for EBUS-guided TBNB in 1299 subjects with lung cancer being evaluated for mediastinal nodal involvement. Notably, only 2 complications occurred in this study (0.15%), affirming the safety and enhanced utility of EBUS in the evaluation of mediastinal lymph nodes. Ernst and colleagues[11] compared EBUS-TBNB to mediastinoscopy, the traditional

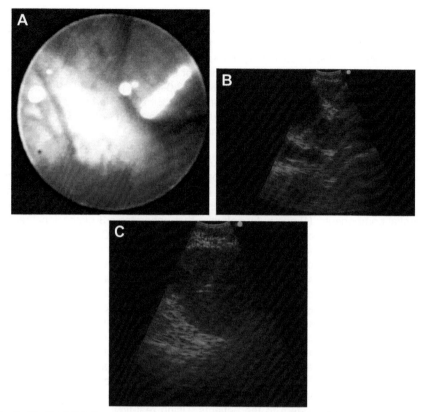

Fig. 5. (A, B, C) EBUS-guided transbronchial needle biopsy of hilar, (B) and right paratracheal lesions in patient with suspected lung cancer.

gold standard for evaluation of mediastinal lymph nodes. In their study, the sensitivity, specificity, and negative predictive value for EBUS-TBNB were 87, 100, and 78%, respectively, compared with 68, 100, and 59%, respectively, for mediastinoscopy. Notably, in the assessment of specific nodal stations, the only area of significant difference was in the subcarinal region where the yield of EBUS-TBNB was superior to mediastinoscopy (98% vs 78%; $P = .007$). A criticism of this study, however, includes the poor outcomes of mediastinoscopy when compared with the results of other large series reported from high-volume thoracic surgical centers.[12,13]

The radial EBUS has further augmented the diagnostic capabilities of the bronchoscopist for evaluating peripheral lesions. With the assistance of a guide sheath, the probe may be advanced beyond the limits visible to a standard bronchoscope. The radial ultrasound is used to localize a pathologic lesion. The ultrasound is then withdrawn and biopsy instruments are advanced through the sheath to sample the area of interest. In a single-center, randomized trial of transbronchial biopsy (TBB) versus EBUS-guided TBB (EBUS-TBB), Paone and colleagues[14] documented a statistically superior sensitivity for the EBUS-TBB cohort (0.79 vs 0.55; $P = .004$). Of note, in subgroup analyses stratifying tumors by size, there was no significant difference noted in sensitivity for lesions greater than 3 cm. For lesions less than 3 cm and those less than 2 cm, EBUS-TBB maintained significant superiority (<3 cm: 0.75 vs 0.31,

P<.001;<2 cm: 0.71 vs 0.23, *P*<.001) Furthermore, significant complications occurred in 10 (8.4%) subjects undergoing TBB, whereas none occurred in the EBUS-TBB group. Kurimoto and colleagues[15] used the radial EBUS probe to evaluate 150 subjects with peripheral pulmonary nodules and achieved a diagnostic yield of 77%. Interestingly, the size of the lesion did not significantly effect the results (<1.0 cm [76%]; 1.0–1.5 cm [76%]; 1.5–2.0 cm [66%]; 2.0–3.0cm [76%]; *P* = .99), supporting the efficacy of this technique for smaller lesions. Similarly, Herth and colleagues[16] achieved a diagnostic yield of 70% in 54 subjects undergoing radial EBUS evaluation of fluoroscopically invisible solitary pulmonary nodules.

Electromagnetic Navigational Bronchoscopy

Electromagnetic navigational bronchoscopy is a promising new technology that provides guidance of a specialized probe beyond the range visible to the bronchoscope, allowing evaluation of peripheral lung lesions. The ENB system consists of 4 essential components: (1) computer software that generates a 3-dimensional reconstruction of the tracheobronchial tree using data obtained from CT scans of the chest; (2) an electromagnetic board connected to the computer containing the planning software that generates a low-dose electromagnetic field; (3) a steerable probe that can be located within the electromagnetic field; and (4) an extended working channel that is initially advanced with the steerable probe and then left in place to maintain the appropriate pathway to the target for diagnostic tools. Before the procedure the bronchoscopist creates a virtual map using the planning software. The procedure subsequently may be performed with conscious sedation or general anesthesia in a room that is specifically designated for the procedure. Patients are positioned on the bronchoscopy table holding the electromagnetic field board and skin sensors are placed. The sensor probe and working channel are advanced through the bronchoscope and reference points identified in the planning stage are located, thus orienting the navigation system to the patients. Using real-time guidance, the sensor probe and working channel are advanced to the target lesion, the working channel is locked into place, and the sensor probe is removed. Various tools, including brushes, needles, and biopsy forceps, may be inserted to obtain diagnostic tissue. Fiducial marks may also be placed to assist with localization of nodules for subsequent therapies, such as stereotactic radiosurgery. The ENB technology may additionally be used for transbronchial needle biopsies of mediastinal lymph nodes and potentially may facilitate delivery of therapeutic devices, such as radiofrequency ablation probes. Fluoroscopy and radial EBUS may also be used to augment imaging capabilities.

The initial investigations of this technology have yielded encouraging results. In the first human trial, Schwarz and colleagues[17] demonstrated a 69% sensitivity rate for the evaluation of peripheral pulmonary lesions. Notably, the size of the lesions ranged from 1.5 to 5 cm and the false negative rate was 30%. More importantly, the investigators documented no adverse events, thus demonstrating the feasibility and safety of this technique. Gildea and colleagues[18] published a series of 58 subjects undergoing ENB revealing a diagnostic yield of 80.3%, which was not statistically different based on lesion size. Of note, the yield for lesions greater than 4.0 cm was 100%. Specific benign diagnoses were made in 14% of cases. Overall the sensitivity for peripheral lesions was 78%. More recently, Eberhardt and colleagues[19] performed a prospective, randomized trial comparing EBUS, ENB, and combined techniques in the evaluation of pulmonary nodules. In the randomized 118 subjects, the diagnostic yield of EBUS and ENB (88%) was significantly higher than that of EBUS alone (69%) or ENB alone (59%). Subgroup analysis based on lesion size, lobar distribution, and

Table 2
Comparison of TBNB, EUS-FNA, and EBUS-TBNB for evaluation of mediastinal lymph nodes in patients with suspected lung cancer

Procedure	Sensitivity (%)	95% Confidence Interval	Negative Predictive Value (%)	95% Confidence Interval
TBNB	36	22–52	78	70–85
EUS-FNA	69	53–82	88	80–93
EBUS-TBNB	69	53–82	88	80–93
EUS-FNA & EBUS TBNB	93	81–99	97	91–99

Data from Wallace MB, Pascual JM, Raimondo M, et al. Minimally invasive endoscopic staging of suspected lung cancer. JAMA 2008;299(5):540–6.

malignant pathology similarly revealed superiority of the combined procedure. No significant bleeding events were encountered and the pneumothorax rate was 6% without significant differences between groups. Of note, the negative predictive value was highest for the combined technique (75% vs 44% for both ENB alone and EBUS alone), thus emphasizing the need for further diagnostic maneuvers when a specific diagnosis is not made.

Endoscopic Ultrasonography

Transesophageal ultrasound-guided fine needle aspiration (EUS-FNA) is complimentary to EBUS in the evaluation of mediastinal lymph nodes as well as in the evaluation of inferior, posterior mediastinal lesions. Lymph node stations accessible to EUS evaluation include left paratracheal (station 4 L), aortoplumonary window (station 5), subcarinal (station 7), paraesophageal (station 8), and inferior pulmonary ligament (station 9). In addition, EUS can be useful for evaluation and biopsy of some liver and adrenal lesions, depending on location and appropriate endocrine evaluation. Curved linear array endoscopes are generally used for real-time needle biopsy and the procedure can be performed under conscious sedation. Studies in subjects with pathologic mediastinal adenopathy either by CT or positron emission tomography (PET) criteria have yielded sensitivity, specificity, negative predictive value, and accuracy of 72% to 100%, 88% to 100%, 39% to 100% and 77% to 100%, respectively.[20] In a direct comparison of traditional-transbronchial needle biopsy (TBNB) with EBUS-TBNB and EUS-FNA, Wallace and colleagues[9] performed all 3 procedures simultaneously on 138 subjects with suspected lung cancer and mediastinal lymph node enlargement. The combination of EBUS-TBNB and EUS-FNA was superior to either method alone (**Table 2**). Vilmann and colleagues[21] additionally revealed a remarkable 100% accuracy using combined modalities for the evaluation of subjects with suspected lung cancer metastases to mediastinal lymph nodes. Notably, the incidence of cancer in this study population was quite high (71%).

Clearly, EBUS, EUS, and ENB have improved the sensitivity and diagnostic yield of the bronchoscopic evaluation of mediastinal lymph nodes and peripheral pulmonary lesions. According to Eberhardt and colleagues[19] these techniques appear to be complimentary and approach the diagnostic yield of more invasive procedures, such as transthoracic needle biopsy or surgical excision. With dissemination of this technology, further studies will be required to validate the results in larger populations and across centers.

SUMMARY

Assessment of the airways and surrounding structures, including the mediastinum and pulmonary parenchyma, has been greatly facilitated by advancements in bronchoscopic techniques, both rigid and flexible. Recent years have seen an explosion in technologies that have revolutionized the ability to visualize, biopsy, or otherwise assess regions of potential pathology within the upper aerodigestive tract and adjacent structures. Although promising, the financial impact and cost effectiveness of these advanced techniques has yet to be determined. In addition, their appropriate implementation will require multidisciplinary input to ascertain that they are used in an effective, efficient, and safe manner relative to other available diagnostic and therapeutic modalities. The surgeon will be well served to learn the technical aspects of the various procedures as well as to keep current regarding outcomes data, including diagnostic yield, accuracy, and complications. Only in this manner will these various technologies and procedures occupy their appropriate place within the surgeon's diagnostic and therapeutic armamentarium.

REFERENCES

1. Marsh BR. Historic development of bronchoesophagology. Otolaryngol Head Neck Surg 1996;114(6):689–716.
2. Conacher ID, Curran E. Local anaesthesia and sedation for rigid bronchoscopy for emergency relief of central airway obstruction. Anaesthesia 2004;59(3):290–2.
3. Lukomsky GI, Ovchinnikov AA, Bilal A. Complications of bronchoscopy: comparison of rigid bronchoscopy under general anesthesia and flexible fiberoptic bronchoscopy under topical anesthesia. Chest 1981;79(3):316–21.
4. Haslam PL, Baughman RP. Report of ERS task force: guidelines for measurement of acellular components and standardization of BAL. Eur Respir J 1999;14(2): 245–8.
5. Schreiber G, McCrory DC. Performance characteristics of different modalities for diagnosis of suspected lung cancer: summary of published evidence. Chest 2003;123(Suppl 1):115S–28S.
6. Baaklini WA, Reinoso MA, Gorin AB, et al. Diagnostic yield of fiberoptic bronchoscopy in evaluating solitary pulmonary nodules. Chest 2000;117(4):1049–54.
7. Heyer CM, Reichelt S, Peters SA, et al. Computed tomography-navigated transthoracic core biopsy of pulmonary lesions: which factors affect diagnostic yield and complication rates? Acad Radiol 2008;15(8):1017–26.
8. Holty JE, Kuschner WG, Gould MK. Accuracy of transbronchial needle aspiration for mediastinal staging of non-small cell lung cancer: a meta-analysis. Thorax 2005;60(11):949–55.
9. Wallace MB, Pascual JM, Raimondo M, et al. Minimally invasive endoscopic staging of suspected lung cancer. JAMA 2008;299(5):540–6.
10. Gu P, Zhao YZ, Jiang LY, et al. Endobronchial ultrasound-guided transbronchial needle aspiration for staging of lung cancer: a systematic review and meta-analysis. Eur J Cancer 2009;45(8):1389–96.
11. Ernst A, Anantham D, Eberhardt R, et al. Diagnosis of mediastinal adenopathy-real-time endobronchial ultrasound guided needle aspiration versus mediastinoscopy. J Thorac Oncol 2008;3(6):577–82.
12. Hammoud ZT, Anderson RC, Meyers BF, et al. The current role of mediastinoscopy in the evaluation of thoracic disease. J Thorac Cardiovasc Surg 1999; 118(5):894–9.

13. Lemaire A, Nikolic I, Petersen T, et al. Nine-year single center experience with cervical mediastinoscopy: complications and false negative rate. Ann Thorac Surg 2006;82(4):1185–9 [discussion: 1189–90].
14. Paone G, Nicastri E, Lucantoni G, et al. Endobronchial ultrasound-driven biopsy in the diagnosis of peripheral lung lesions. Chest 2005;128(5):3551–7.
15. Kurimoto N, Miyazawa T, Okimasa S, et al. Endobronchial ultrasonography using a guide sheath increases the ability to diagnose peripheral pulmonary lesions endoscopically. Chest 2004;126(3):959–65.
16. Herth FJ, Eberhardt R, Becker HD, et al. Endobronchial ultrasound-guided transbronchial lung biopsy in fluoroscopically invisible solitary pulmonary nodules: a prospective trial. Chest 2006;129(1):147–50.
17. Schwarz Y, Greif J, Becker HD, et al. Real-time electromagnetic navigation bronchoscopy to peripheral lung lesions using overlaid CT images: the first human study. Chest 2006;129(4):988–94.
18. Gildea TR, Mazzone PJ, Karnak D, et al. Electromagnetic navigation diagnostic bronchoscopy: a prospective study. Am J Respir Crit Care Med 2006;174(9): 982–9.
19. Eberhardt R, Anantham D, Ernst A, et al. Multimodality bronchoscopic diagnosis of peripheral lung lesions: a randomized controlled trial. Am J Respir Crit Care Med 2007;176(1):36–41.
20. Herth FJ, Ernst A, Eberhardt R, et al. Endobronchial ultrasound-guided transbronchial needle aspiration of lymph nodes in the radiologically normal mediastinum. Eur Respir J 2006;28(5):910–4.
21. Vilmann P, Krasnik M, Larsen SS, et al. Transesophageal endoscopic ultrasound-guided fine-needle aspiration (EUS-FNA) and endobronchial ultrasound-guided transbronchial needle aspiration (EBUS-TBNA) biopsy: a combined approach in the evaluation of mediastinal lesions. Endoscopy 2005;37(9):833–9.

The Compromised Airway: Tumors, Strictures, and Tracheomalacia

Henning A. Gaissert, MD[a],*, James Burns, MD[b]

KEYWORDS

- Tracheomalacia • Acute airway obstruction
- Upper airway tumors • Intubation injury

This article reviews the presentation, causes, and interventions for a select group of intrinsic airway disorders involving larynx and trachea. These disorders have in common the dual surgical aspects of managing acute airway obstruction and selecting the definitive treatment of the underlying cause. The anatomic region from the larynx to the carina is discussed, keeping in mind that sometimes more distal obstruction at the level of one (after pneumonectomy) or both mainstem bronchi may also lead to asphyxiation. The discussion, however, does not provide an exhaustive review of all causes of airway obstruction; the authors concentrate on tumors and strictures in the larynx and trachea and on tracheomalacia, excluding oropharyngeal disorders such as sleep apnea, extrinsic disease secondarily impairing respiration, and small airway diseases. Although the compromised airway is often a dramatic surgical emergency, slowly evolving symptoms may for many months remain unrecognized and be indeed misdiagnosed as parenchymal lung disease, for example as adult onset of asthma. The urgency of presentation and degree of respiratory compensation in the presence of significant stenosis is therefore variable and depends on location, rate of progression, and specific cause of obstruction. When considering intrinsic obstruction of the larynx and trachea, the vast majority of patients belong to a few categories of disease: metastatic carcinoma, primary tumors of the airway, strictures after endotracheal intubation or mechanical ventilation, and inflammatory strictures unrelated to instrumentation of the airway. The authors also discuss the surgical management of dynamic

---

[a] Division of Thoracic and Laryngeal Surgery, Massachusetts General Hospital, Department of Surgery, Harvard Medical School, Boston, MA, USA
[b] Division of Thoracic and Laryngeal Surgery, Massachusetts General Hospital, Harvard Medical School, Boston, MA, USA
* Corresponding author. Division of Thoracic Surgery, Massachusetts General Hospital, Blake 1570, 55 Fruit St, Boston, MA 02114.
E-mail address: hgaissert@partners.org

Surg Clin N Am 90 (2010) 1065–1089
doi:10.1016/j.suc.2010.06.004
0039-6109/10/$ – see front matter © 2010 Elsevier Inc. All rights reserved.

surgical.theclinics.com

expiratory collapse of the trachea associated with emphysema, commonly called tracheomalacia.

The surgeon consulted for acute airway obstruction must order his or her[a] thoughts quickly, assemble a team, and devise a treatment plan with more than one contingency in mind. Conversely, a patient presenting with minor hemoptysis or gradual progression of breathing difficulties in chronic obstruction permits the systematic evaluation of a cause before the surgeon commits to intervention. The common principle in the management of acute airway obstruction is to support the awake, spontaneously breathing patient until the intervention is prepared, to select an immediate intervention that does not compromise the chances for success of definitive therapy, and to embark on definitive therapy only when circumstances are favorable and success is likely. Because of their importance, these two components are discussed repeatedly throughout this article. In considering the management of acute airway obstruction the authors remain conscious that a majority of readers may be general surgeons unfamiliar with rigid bronchoscopy, yet seeking guidance on how to obtain a secure airway.

DIMENSIONS OF THE NORMAL AIRWAY

The adult airway from the true vocal cords to the carina measures approximately 13 to 15 cm. The first 2 cm to the cricoid cartilage form the subglottic space. From the lower edge of the cricoid to the carinal spur, the trachea therefore measures 11 to 13 cm in length. The narrowest plane of the upper airway is located at the level of the vocal cords. The area of opening at the glottic level during inspiration in healthy adults is approximately 130 mm^2 with an interarytenoid distance of 12 mm.[1] The shape of the normal trachea varies from horseshoe to oval and is influenced by the impression of the aortic arch. The horseshoe shape is maintained by the cartilaginous skeleton and the smooth muscle in the membranous portion. The normal adult diameter varies between 11 and 25 mm depending on patient size and tracheal level, usually being longer in the anteroposterior dimension. The two extremes of the upper airway are relatively fixed, providing points of endoscopic reference to relate abnormal findings in distance; describing a lesion as merely "subglottic" has little value because this location is shared by the rest of the respiratory system. The fixation of these 2 points creates the original challenge in tracheal resection because even surgical release maneuvers of larynx or carina add only limited length to the trachea and reduce, but do not prevent, anastomotic tension. Because tracheal length limits the options for surgical reconstruction, maximal preservation of normal tracheal wall must be foremost in the mind of the surgeon.

VASCULAR SUPPLY OF THE TRACHEA

In careful autopsy studies, Salassa and colleagues[2] described the arterial blood supply of the trachea. There are several important findings. Multiple small arteries, originating as branches of the supreme intercostal, the inferior thyroid, the internal thoracic, the phrenic, and the bronchial arteries, supply longitudinal arcades on either side of the trachea. This blood supply is shared with the esophagus, meaning that resection of the esophagus severely impairs, indeed renders unlikely, the healing of

---

[a] There is no single correct possessive pronoun because in some years more than 50% of general surgical residents at Massachusetts General Hospital [MGH] are women.

tracheal anastomoses. The blood supply of the trachea is segmental; excessive surgical mobilization of tracheal ends extending for more than 1 to 2 cm, and therefore risks anastomotic ischemia and dehiscence. The segmental arteries supply a submucosal plexus that in turn is the only source of blood to the semilunar cartilages. Denuded cartilage, for example, by pressure from a tracheal tube cuff, becomes necrotic and sloughs off. Vascularity is such a prominent concern because tracheal anastomoses are subjected to amounts of tension unlike that seen after intestinal or bronchial sleeve resection. Any arterial compromise, including the microangiopathies associated with diabetes mellitus and radiation, is thus reflected in a higher anastomotic failure rate.[3]

PRESENTATION

The presence of airway obstruction is either overt and immediately life-threatening or obscure and not clearly attributed to the airway. Disregarding trauma, any acute obstruction may have been present for weeks, months, or years; often patients are surprisingly well adapted for a time to subglottic or tracheal high-grade narrowing, in particular if they pursue a sedentary lifestyle. When obstructive symptoms appear at rest, the airway cross section usually has narrowed to less than 30% of normal, equivalent to an airway diameter of 5 to 6 mm. In this situation, thick respiratory secretions may lead to sudden, complete obstruction and asphyxiation. Inspiratory airway obstruction is often associated with fixed obstruction of the larynx and upper trachea, whereas expiratory symptoms are more common in the dynamic collapse of tracheomalacia and lower airway obstruction. Any patient with a history of endotracheal intubation who presents with dyspnea, wheezing, or stridor must be assumed to have postintubation stenosis until proved otherwise. Because these patients may resume physical activity only gradually after recovery from their illness, loss of muscle strength may mask their diagnosis. A systemic disease may provide important clues. Patients with chronic obstructive lung disease may develop tracheomalacia; polychondritis apparent from deformed nasal and auricular cartilage may present in the airways; a history of tuberculosis should raise the suspicion of tracheobronchial involvement. Patients with rheumatoid arthritis may develop cricoarytenoid joint fixation with bilateral vocal fold immobility. Most, but not all, forms of malignant obstruction evolve over a course of less than 6 months. It is common for shortness of breath in bronchogenic malignancy to progress rapidly over 1 to 3 months, as it is associated with a general decline. Dyspnea associated with laryngeal malignancies is often accompanied by hoarseness, dysphagia or odynophagia, and referred otalgia.

RADIOGRAPHIC EVALUATION

In tracheal obstructive disease, a plain film of the chest often shows clear lungs; an abnormal tracheal air column, though often overlooked, may provide an important clue. Conversely, a unilateral lung mass suggests malignant tracheal obstruction. The patient with tracheomalacia, by contrast, often demonstrates hyperinflation resulting from chronic obstructive pulmonary disease, and may have a normal air column. Standard linear 2-dimensional tomography, though highly accurate in demonstrating the length of a tracheal lesion, has ceased to be available in many hospitals. The information provided by computed tomography (CT) and particularly multidetector computed tomography (MDCT) make these two imaging modalities indispensable in the evaluation of airway obstruction unless asphyxiation is imminent. MDCT acquires volumetric data in a single breath-hold, minimizing respiratory and cardiac motion artifacts; it integrates axial images and multiplanar reformats with

3-dimensional rendering and allows precise delineation of the location, length, and mural depth of tracheal pathology.[4] This information is useful to gauge the length of a high-grade stenosis not previously traversed with the bronchoscope, to evaluate the extrinsic component and length of a tracheal tumor or, with dynamic imaging of inspiration and expiration in patients with tracheomalacia, to detect respiratory changes in tracheal diameter. **Fig. 1** demonstrates an example of MDCT in a primary tracheal tumor.

BRONCHOSCOPY

The endoscopic assessment of the cause and extent of airway obstruction is indispensable to locate and measure the narrowing, to relieve symptoms, and to plan treatment. The diagnosis infers that the physiologic mechanisms of respiratory compensation are already impaired or nearly exhausted. Thus, careful preparation of this procedure is critical to prevent irretrievable loss of airway and death of the patient. Such preparation entails the assembly of a team consisting of anesthesiologist and surgeon and their support personnel, the communication among members of the team of a procedural plan with consideration of potential risks and their

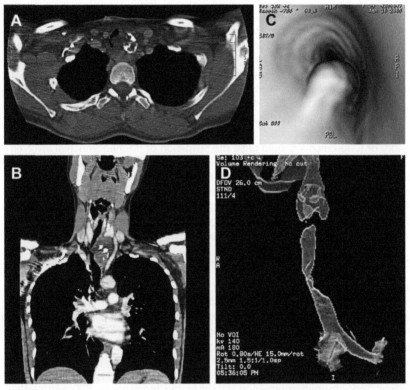

Fig. 1. Multidetector computed tomography of a 6.5-cm long adenoid cystic carcinoma of the trachea. (*A*) Standard cross-sectional image of high-grade obstruction. (*B*) Coronal cut. (*C*) Virtual bronchoscopic image of high-grade obstruction. (*D*) Axial outline of tracheal lumen. Note that panels *C* and *D* do not provide information about tracheal wall or tumor thickness.

management, the assembly and testing for proper function of all necessary equipment for rigid and fiberoptic bronchoscopy in the procedure room, and the preparation for a surgical airway. Anesthetist and surgeon have a shared and indivisible responsibility for the patient during bronchoscopy; plans for muscle relaxation and access to the airway must be coordinated because neither medical nor legal responsibility can easily be separated. Maintaining spontaneous respiration is highly desirable as long as the airway is not secure, and inhalation agents nonirritating to the airway such as Halothane (2-bromo-2-chloro-1,1,1-trifluoroethane) or Sevoflurane (2,2,2-trifluoro-1-[trifluoromethyl]ethyl fluoromethyl ether) are therefore preferred for induction. Awake interventions are questionable when obstruction is acute; the added stress increases oxygen consumption and may lead to acute respiratory decompensation.

LARYNGOSCOPY

Visualization of the larynx in patients suspected of having obstruction or other pathology at the laryngeal level can often be done indirectly in the office setting using a mirror or endoscope. Various flexible (transnasal) and rigid (transoral) endoscopes are available, with flexible scopes potentially able to provide additional information about the subglottis and upper trachea in patients who tolerate passage of the scope through the vocal folds. These systems are easily adapted to video recording equipment for documentation of lesions, degree of mucosal inflammation, vocal fold mobility, and airway patency. Care is first taken to ensure that patients are not in an extreme airway-compromised condition, and that they can tolerate an office-based examination.

Direct laryngoscopy under general anesthesia is helpful in determining cricoarytenoid joint mobility, in staging laryngeal tumors and determining resectability of benign and malignant laryngeal lesions, and in assessing airway caliber at the glottic level. Large glottiscopes can often easily access and adequately expose the laryngeal inlet for subsequent placement of rigid telescopes to assess the remaining airway. Similar to bronchoscopy, direct laryngoscopy requires confidence and close cooperation between the surgeon and the anesthesiologist.

Acute Obstruction and the General Surgeon

A surgeon unfamiliar with the rigid ventilating bronchoscope is bereft of the most versatile diagnostic and interventional tool for the trachea. With a flexible, fiberoptic bronchoscope the surgeon may at least inspect the uppermost extent of obstruction, thus allowing a visual distinction between benign and malignant cause, but this endoscope is unsuitable for critical airway obstruction because passage across the obstruction exacerbates symptoms akin to the cork closing the bottle. Although fiberoptic bronchoscopy permits biopsy and the application of a laser beam to relieve obstruction, the endoscopist is liable to lose the airway if bleeding occurs or tumor fragments fall into the lumen. Self-expanding metal or plastic airway stents often lead to immediate impressive improvement of airway diameter and symptoms; however, their uncritical use in benign strictures or in resectable tumors may limit surgical options, has been shown to result in complications,[5] and has produced a Food and Drug Administration advisory regarding their indications.[6] Benign tracheobronchial strictures should not be palliated with self-expanding stents because these stents extend the injury and may lead to wire fracture, airway perforation, or vascular fistula.

The choice between airway stent, endotracheal intubation, and tracheostomy in the acute setting depends on individual circumstances. Clearly unresectable tumors or obstruction caused by metastatic lymph nodes are appropriately treated with self-expanding stents. In an emergency, extrinsic obstruction or resectable tumors may be managed with endotracheal intubation for later referral to a specialized center; a selection of endotracheal tubes in varying sizes, from 4 mm upwards, should be available. Temporizing management of a recognized postintubation tracheal stricture may consist in reopening the tracheal stoma or performing a new tracheostomy through the stenotic, diseased trachea; the tracheal stoma should not use up additional length of normal trachea needed for later reconstruction.

Acute Obstruction and the Thoracic Surgeon

A rigid ventilating bronchoscope is the best tool to investigate acute or chronic airway obstruction. If a stricture is localized within the larynx, suspension laryngoscopy should precede examination of the trachea. Securing the laryngoscope with a suspension apparatus allows for controlled assessment of the laryngeal structures, including palpation of the cricoarytenoid joints to differentiate between joint fixation and denervation in patients with known or suspected vocal fold immobility. The entire airway is inspected during the examination to assess the length of normal relative to diseased trachea. Measurements are obtained by determining the distance between the patient's upper incisors and markings on the metal endoscope at various landmarks such as carina, lower and upper end of stricture or tumor, tracheal stoma, cricoid ring, and vocal cords.

If postintubation injury is suspected, bronchoscopic dilatation may precede attempts at tracheostomy or immediate tracheal resection. Tracheal dilatation alone is unlikely to produce prolonged palliation of breathing but sometimes provides time to plan for definitive therapy. The rigid endoscope permits dilatation under controlled conditions, maintaining ventilation of both lungs. Jackson-type bronchoscopes are ideally suited to dilatation because they possess a blunt, rounded tip. The adult sizes are 7, 8, and 9 mm, and shorter pediatric endoscopes of the sizes 4, 5, and 6 mm are available. The tip of the rigid bronchoscope is gently introduced into the stricture in a rotatory motion. Tight strictures less than 6 mm in diameter are dilated with esophageal Jackson dilators (Pilling Surgical Inc, Research Triangle Park, NC, USA) inserted through an adult bronchoscope. Serial dilatation with advancing sizes of dilators and bronchoscopes enlarges the diameter gradually.

In the evaluation of tumors, the surgeon should first decide whether tracheal resection is at all realistic. If the tracheal obstruction is metastatic, the rigid endoscope is used to resect the mass as needed to immediately enlarge the lumen.[7] External beam radiation or brachytherapy may later provide more definitive palliation. Tumor is cored out by directing the blunt tip of the endoscope parallel to the tracheal wall to prevent injury to residual cartilage or membranous portion. The resulting tumor fragments are removed with the biopsy forceps, and bleeding is controlled either with dilute epinephrine solution (epinephrine 1:1000 1 mL in 19 mL saline) or by placing the wall of the endoscope against the bleeding surface. While not an essential tool, a laser may also be used to enlarge the lumen. Endoscopic resection to enlarge the airway lumen before tracheal resection is used sparingly, if at all, and any injury to the remaining length of normal trachea must be painstakingly avoided.

SPECIFIC DISEASES
Laryngeal Obstruction

In the adult population laryngeal neoplasms rarely present with acute airway obstruction but are often suspected, based on other aerodigestive symptoms such as hoarseness, throat tightness, dysphagia, odynophagia, referred otalgia or, in the case of malignancy, appearance of a palpable neck mass. However, benign and malignant neoplasms have the potential to cause laryngeal obstruction either directly by growing into the airway lumen or indirectly by compromising function of the recurrent laryngeal nerves or the cricoarytenoid joint, leading to vocal fold immobility. Bilateral vocal fold immobility causes glottic obstruction with the vocal folds often resting in a near-closed position, whereas unilateral vocal fold immobility rarely presents with obstructive symptoms. Acute infections such as laryngotracheobronchitis and epiglottitis, and inflammatory conditions such as allergic angioedema often present with rapidly progressing airway distress and represent true airway emergencies.

The most common benign neoplasm causing laryngeal obstruction is recurrent respiratory papillomatosis associated with human papilloma virus infection. This epithelial-trophic virus produces exophytic warty growths on vocal folds that recur often after treatment. These lesions most often disrupt phonation, but the disease can progress to involve supraglottic and subglottic areas and cause airway obstructive symptoms. Treatment involves endoscopic ablation of the papillomatous growths with emphasis toward preservation of the underlying vocal fold layered microstructure that is critical for maintaining phonation. After initially treating papilloma with pulsed-KTP laser photoangiolysis in the operating room under general anesthesia, most patients tolerate ablation of recurrent disease with office-based photoangiolysis under local anesthesia.[8,9]

More than 90% of primary malignant laryngeal tumors are squamous cell carcinomas. Patients presenting with these lesions can develop significant airway obstruction either from the burden of disease or in response to treatment, such as the development of acute swelling during chemoradiation therapy. Initial management of laryngeal carcinoma includes direct laryngoscopy for tumor staging and a multidisciplinary approach to treatment planning that includes optimal surgical treatment, appropriate consideration of adjuvant therapies such as chemoradiation, and an assessment of the impact of loss of voice and swallowing functions in a particular patient. Acute airway management includes laser debulking of obstructive tumors and placement of a tracheotomy if needed. Repeat laryngoscopy in patients undergoing radiation therapy for laryngeal cancer is prudent to detect those patients who are developing edema and possible airway compromise. Contemporary management of most early (T1, T2) laryngeal malignancies includes endoscopic surgical excision with external approaches such as extensive partial and total laryngectomies reserved for more advanced disease.[10,11]

Bilateral vocal fold immobility most often is the iatrogenic result of neck surgery such as thyroidectomy, but this condition can also develop from injury or other disease process impinging the vagus or recurrent laryngeal nerves anywhere from the brainstem to the point of entry into the larynx. Evaluation beyond a thorough otolaryngologic examination therefore includes a CT scan of head, neck, and chest with contrast to assess the entire course of the recurrent laryngeal nerve from the skull base to the superior mediastinum. These patients have significantly compromised airways, as there is often no more than a 4 to 6 mm opening at the glottic level. Even when well compensated the tenuous nature of the airway must be appreciated, as the slightest degree of glottic swelling associated with a viral upper respiratory infection or allergy can cause complete or near-complete airway obstruction. Airway management includes endoscopic surgical strategies to open the posterior glottic aperture, such as partial arytenoidectomy and suture lateralization of the vocal cord.[12]

Malignant Tracheal Obstruction

Airway obstruction due to tumor erosion into mainstem bronchi, carina, or trachea often requires palliative intervention. Lung, laryngeal, or esophageal cancer are common thoracic malignancies, and their metastatic peritracheal lymph nodes regularly invade the tracheal lumen. The diagnosis is rarely a challenge because CT findings describe precisely the origin of obstruction. The role of the surgeon is to provide a diagnosis and to relieve obstruction as explained in the section on bronchoscopy. Except for carcinomas of the thyroid, palliative resection is rarely employed. As long as at least one recurrent laryngeal nerve is preserved, combined resection of thyroid and trachea with tracheal or laryngotracheal reconstruction effectively controls hemoptysis and restores a normal tracheal lumen[13]; many of these patients experience prolonged, though not disease-free survival. In patients with tumors other than thyroid carcinoma, survival after diagnosis of malignant tracheal obstruction is short, due to rapid systemic progression of disease.

Primary Tracheal Tumors

Malignant tracheal obstruction is common whereas primary tracheal tumors are rare. The difference in incidence to primary tumors is striking and according to some estimates, metastatic lesions exceed primary tumors of the trachea by a factor of 1000.[14] A metastatic malignancy should therefore be assumed unless additional findings point to primary disease. The presence of a primary tumor is suggested by absence of lung masses except those consistent with pulmonary metastases of tracheal carcinoma, absence of extensive mediastinal or hilar lymph node enlargement, and absence of distant metastasis. The challenge consists of finding the few primary tumors among the many that are not.

An overwhelming majority of remaining primary tumors are malignant, even when one excludes from this calculation the 2 most common tracheal cancers, squamous cell and adenoid cystic carcinoma. The remaining neoplasms consist of diverse lesions, among them mucoepidermoid carcinoma, nonsquamous carcinoma, sarcoma, and carcinoid tumors. In a large clinical series including resected and unresectable primary tracheal tumors, malignant lesions predominated (**Table 1**). The expectation of malignant primary neoplasms informs also the selection of therapy. Because less than 10% of tumors in a single-institution series were benign[15] and most tumors grow in a transmural manner, one may conclude that subtotal removal by endobronchial techniques does not constitute adequate treatment of a tracheal tumor because complete resection cannot be confirmed.

Presentation

Diagnostic delay is the rule, on average amounting to 12 months in the MGH series. **Fig. 2** shows that the duration of this delay is related to the type of tumor; except for adenoid cystic carcinoma, benign and low-grade malignant tumors have a longer delay than high-grade malignancies. The 2 most common tracheal tumors, squamous and adenoid cystic carcinoma, have important differences in the type of symptoms, as shown in **Table 2**.

Evaluation

The evaluation of the primary tracheal tumor consists of an assessment of local disease, histologic confirmation, and clinical staging of regional and distant disease. While local assessment is facilitated by a precise, thin-section MDCT aided by sagittal and coronal reconstruction, as noted earlier, bronchoscopy under general anesthesia

Table 1 Primary tracheal tumors	
Malignant Lesions	**No. of Patients**
Adenoid cystic carcinoma	135
Squamous cell carcinoma	135
Carcinoids:	11
Typical	10
Atypical	1
Lymphoma	2
Melanoma	1
Mucoepidermoid carcinoma	14
Nonsquamous carcinoma	15
Small cell carcinoma	5
Adenocarcinoma	4
Large cell carcinoma	4
Adenosquamous carcinoma	2
Sarcoma	13
Spindle cell sarcoma	6
Chondrosarcoma	3
Leiomyosarcoma	1
Carcinosarcoma (pseudosarcoma)	1
Invasive fibrous tumor	1
Malignant fibrous histiocytoma	1
All malignant	*326*
Benign Lesions	
Capillary hemangioma	1
Chondroblastoma	1
Chondroma	2
Fibrous histiocytoma	1
Glomus tumor	1
Granular cell tumor	2
Hamartoma	2
Hemangiomatous malformation of mediastinum	1
Inflammatory pseudotumor (plasma cell granuloma)	1
Leiomyoma	3
Neurogenic tumor	4
Schwannoma	1
Plexiform neurofibroma	1
Peripheral nerve sheath tumor	1
Atypical schwannoma	1
Paraganglioma	1
Pleomorphic adenoma	3
Pyogenic granuloma	1
Squamous papillomas	9
Multiple	5
Solitary	4
Vascular tumor of borderline malignancy	1
All benign	*34*
Total	360

The histologic diagnosis of 360 tracheal tumors in 357 patients seen over more than 40 years at Massachusetts General Hospital (MGH). Malignant tumors predominate; nonsquamous bronchogenic carcinomas are rare. Three patients had 2 tumors of different histology. As reported in Refs.[15,18]

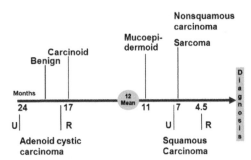

Fig. 2. Average duration of symptoms in patients with primary tracheal tumors. The duration is expressed in months as a distance from diagnosis along a horizontal axis. Mean delay was 12 months. The 2 most common primary carcinomas, squamous and adenoid cystic carcinoma, are separated into unresectable (U) and resected (R) patients.

provides essential information about the length of diseased and uninvolved trachea. Where available, endobronchial ultrasonography may provide additional information about tracheal wall thickness and extent of extrinsic tumor, though endosonography has not been shown to improve staging.

Biopsy is not always obligatory before resection; short, obstructive lesions can be resected without biopsy, but a histologic diagnosis in more extensive tumors may influence the judgment on whether a primary tumor is present and resectable. Whereas the pathologic interpretation is often straightforward, the diagnosis of adenoid cystic carcinoma is sometimes difficult where this tumor type is rarely seen. How else would one explain the frequency of the extremely uncommon tracheal adenocarcinoma exceeding 10% in epidemiologic studies,[16,17] if not by misdiagnosis of adenoid cystic carcinoma or metastatic disease? A diagnosis of adenocarcinoma should be confirmed by an experienced pathologist and accompanied by radiographic review to precisely separate primary from metastatic lesions.

Clinical evaluation for distant disease consists of standard radiographic studies, including combined computed and positron emission tomography (CT-PET) and CT or magnetic resonance imaging of the brain. In a referral center, less than 10% of all patients with tracheal tumors, selected for assumed resectability, were found to have metastatic disease.[18] The proportion of distant disease is expected to be much higher in unselected patients, particularly those with squamous cell carcinoma, and justifies a detailed metastatic survey. The value of PET depends on the tumor type and grade; whereas squamous cell carcinomas exhibit uniformly high uptake, the avidity on PET of adenoid cystic or mucoepidermoid carcinoma depends on their degree of differentiation.[19]

Therapy
Given the immediate proximity to important vascular structures and lymphatic channels, the very fact that any of these central tumors are resectable at all may seem astonishing. Local invasion of aorta, innominate artery, superior vena cava, or pulmonary artery is uncommon, and esophageal invasion can often be excised by resection of the muscle layer alone or resection of part of the esophageal circumference; either technique preserves the original swallowing conduit. The mobile excursion of the trachea relative to the surrounding mediastinal structures may resist fixation by tumor early in the natural history. The limited rate of lymph node metastasis and distant disease at the time of resection is perhaps best understood when considering the

Table 2
Characteristics and comorbidity in patients with squamous and adenoid cystic carcinoma

	ACC	SCC	χ^2 P Value
Sex			
Female	53%	32%	.004
Male	46%	68%	
Mean age (median), years	49 (47)	61 (62)	
Comorbidities (%)			
Smoker	45	89	<.001
Hypertension	17	29	.02
EtOH use	5	18	<.001
Past VII	2	13	.001
Diabetes mellitus	2	12	.002
Steroid use	7	7	.812
Angina	3	6	.238
Arrhythmia	3	5	.356
Prior stroke	2	3	.702
Prior cancers (%)			
Lung	1	15	<.0001
Larynx	0	7	.001
Head and neck	0	4	.024
Colon	1	1	.562
Prostate	1	1	.562
Oropharynx	0	1	.156
Other	0	7	.001
Symptoms (%)			
Dyspnea	65	50	.014
Cough	55	52	.626
Hemoptysis	29	60	<.001
Wheeze	44	27	.003
Stridor	21	27	.200
Hoarseness	10	13	.495
Dysphagia	7	7	.812
Fever	7	4	.184
Other	12	14	.495

Abbreviations: ACC, adenoid cystic carcinoma; SCC, squamous cell carcinoma; EtOH, alcohol; MI, myocardial infarction.
Data from Gaissert HA, Grillo HC, Shadmehr MB, et al. Long-term survival after resection of primary adenoid cystic and squamous cell carcinoma of the trachea and carina. Ann Thorac Surg 2004;78:1889–97.

size of resected tumors. The mean length of resected trachea at MGH in adenoid cystic carcinoma was 3.2 cm and in squamous cell carcinoma, 2.4 cm.[18] Therefore, inferring from the association of tumor mass and lymph node metastasis in broncho-genic carcinoma, neither lymph node spread nor dissemination of disease should be common by the time obstructive symptoms lead to the diagnosis of a resectable tracheal tumor.

For the patient in respiratory distress, rapid relief is provided by endobronchial debulking as described earlier. Endobronchial laser may also be used for this purpose, but airway stenting is undesirable because of the additional injury inflicted by the stent on the tracheal wall.

The selection of definitive therapy proceeds from a determination of resectability. There is now enough evidence showing the superior long-term outcome of segmental tracheal resection in terms of survival and function.[18,20] Resection restores a normal airway lumen and does not preclude additional postoperative therapy, neither radiation nor chemotherapy. In contrast, neoadjuvant chemotherapy has not been demonstrated to increase survival, and preoperative radiotherapy exponentially increases the risk of anastomotic dehiscence. The decision to resect is influenced by tumor length, neck mobility, comorbid factors, and age. There is no universally applicable limit for the maximum resectable length, although resection of more than half of the trachea rarely succeeds. The longer the tumor, the greater should be the emphasis on accurate surgical judgment. At present, the use of prosthetic or biologic forms of tracheal replacement is not clinically established, but replacement may become available in the future. When longer-term palliation is sought, the authors prefer the silicone T-tube.

The close spatial relationships in the mediastinum do not allow radical resection in a radial plane, while limited tracheal length and mobility restrict the taking of margins along the tracheal axis. So constrained, doubts must arise regarding the completeness of any tracheal resection for tumor. Indeed, margins are often close or microscopically positive in resections for adenoid cystic carcinoma, the archetypical surgical challenge due to its extensive submucosal spread at the time of diagnosis. In the MGH series, 59% of resections for adenoid cystic carcinoma resulted in positive margins at either tracheal cut end or along the soft tissue.[18] In a more complete follow-up of adenoid cystic carcinoma, patients with microscopically positive airway margins after resection did worse than those with negative tracheal margins but had superior survival to patients with unresectable disease, as shown in **Fig. 3**.[21] Because most tracheal carcinomas extend through the tracheal wall the tumor is often close to the soft tissue surface, without invasion into adjacent structures. The frequent proximity of tumor to the radial margin led early on to the recommendation for postoperative radiotherapy that today is part of standard therapy. **Table 3** shows the influence of tumor depth and lymphatic invasion on survival after resection of squamous cell carcinoma, based on individual pathologic review of resected squamous cell carcinoma.[22] Although extension beyond the tracheal wall and lymphatic invasion lower survival, their mere presence should not preempt surgical therapy. Despite unfavorable anatomic relationships, the existing evidence supports the preference for resection.

Patients in whom a primary tracheal anastomosis after tumor resection is judged impossible, those with disease locally invasive into organs other than the esophagus, and those with metastatic disease are considered unresectable. These patients are candidates for primary radiation or radiochemotherapy to palliate breathing. Their survival is short in the case of high-grade bronchogenic carcinoma and sarcoma, but adenoid cystic carcinoma has a slower rate of progression and often responds to radiation with prolonged survival despite the evolution of metastatic disease. The value of palliative resection for the individual patient with metastatic adenoid cystic carcinoma must be questioned.

The fate of the anastomosis is the primary determinant of operative success in strictly tracheal resections. There is no generally valid answer as to how much trachea is safely resectable. Instead, several variables are considered: patient age, mobility of the neck, body weight and build, and endoscopically determined length of lesion. A composite assessment of the first 3 factors indicates how high the trachea will rise

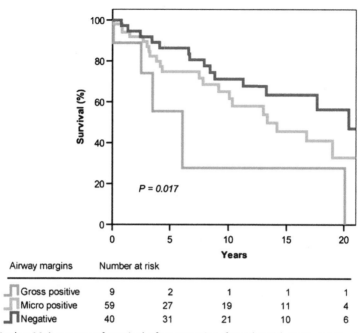

Fig. 3. Kaplan-Meier curve of survival after resection for adenoid cystic carcinoma of the trachea. There is separation of survival of patients with microscopically positive tracheal margin from both negative and grossly positive margins. (*Data from* Honings J, Gaissert HA, Weinberg AC, et al. Prognostic value of pathologic characteristics and resection margins in tracheal adenoid cystic carcinoma. Eur J Cardiothorac Surg, 2010;37:1438–44.)

out of the chest during maximal neck extension and whether complete mobilization of the trachea together with surgical release maneuvers would add sufficient length for safe reconstruction; these considerations will need to be balanced with the antici-pated length of resection. Planned resections of less than 4 cm of trachea will almost always be tolerated, unless incomplete mobilization or fixed cervical kyphosis raises anastomotic tension. Carinal resections have further risks related to an additional anastomosis or major pulmonary resection. The greater complexity is reflected in a higher operative mortality (tracheal resection 3.9%, carinal resection 16%) in the MGH series.[18] The results of 900 tracheal resections for various indications were analyzed for factors predicting anastomotic complications.[3] In stepwise analysis these risk factors were reoperation, diabetes, resection of more than 4 cm of trachea, laryngotracheal resection, young age, and the presence of a tracheostomy at the time of resection. **Fig. 1** shows the increase of anastomotic complications as a function of resected tracheal length. Tumor as the indication for resection, by contrast, did not predict anastomotic failure. These observations emphasize the importance of a well-executed first tracheal resection.

While complete mediastinal lymph node dissection appears desirable for precise staging, tracheal devascularization should be assumed after radical removal of peri-tracheal lymph nodes; confidence may be placed in either staging or healing, but not both. The segmental tracheal blood vessels in the vicinity of peritracheal lymph nodes must be preserved. While lymph nodes immediately adjacent to tumor are often part of the specimen, systematic nodal staging is undesirable. Confirmed lymph node

Table 3
Survival according to depth of tracheal wall invasion and lymphatic invasion in squamous cell carcinoma

Pathologic Subgroup	No.	No. (%)	Mean Survival (Years)	P Value	Survival (%) 5-Year	10-Year
Depth of Invasion				.001		
Carcinoma in situ	2	3.4	Not available		100	100
Infiltrating lamina propria	5	8.5	7.6		75	25
Abutting or extending between cartilage	14	23.7	6.0		50	25
Invading beyond cartilage	11	18.6	7.1		50	38
Invading peritracheal fibroadipose tissue	16	27.1	7.7		53	31
Abutting soft tissue resection margin	6	10.2	2.1			
Invading into thyroid gland	5	8.5	1.4		0	
Lymphatic Invasion[a]				.049		
Yes	22	37.3	4.6		24	24
No	37	62.7	7.6		60	31
Overall	59	100.0	6.5		46	27

Note steep decline in survival once tumor extends to soft tissue margin or invades the thyroid.
[a] Lymphatic invasion proved by either positive lymph node biopsy or lymphatic invasion on histologic examination.

Data from Honings J, Gaissert HA, Ruangchira-Urai R, et al. Pathologic characteristics of resected squamous cell carcinoma of the trachea: prognostic factors based on an analysis of 59 cases. Virchows Arch 2009;455:423–9.

metastasis lowers long-term survival; indeed survival beyond 10 years in lymph node–positive adenoid cystic carcinoma was not observed at MGH.

The evidence for adjuvant therapy is incomplete and circumstantial. The recommendation for additional local therapy is based on the compromised completeness of almost all resections for intermediate or high-grade malignant tumors. Low-grade tumors such as carcinoid tumor or well-differentiated mucoepidermoid carcinoma do not receive radiation. At MGH, every patient with aggressive malignancy who has completed recovery with an intact tracheal anastomosis receives mediastinal radiation with a dose of 54 Gy. Some patients treated elsewhere have received higher doses. Radiotherapy should be delayed if there are concerns about the anastomosis, and treatment is usually not started for 2 months after surgery.

Follow-up and results
Continued follow-up of these patients has the purpose of monitoring for locoregional and distant recurrence as well as second primary cancers. In the MGH series, 27 of 135 patients with squamous cell carcinomas of the trachea had prior carcinomas of the lung, head, or neck. Second primary tumors therefore threaten these patients in the future. Regular surveillance CT and bronchoscopy should be offered to all patients to diagnose locoregional recurrence early, even though second resections for recurrent tumor would rarely be considered.

The mean survival of resected squamous cell carcinoma was 38 months and that of unresectable tumors 8.8 months. The 5-year survival of squamous cell carcinoma was 39% after resection and 7.3% from the time of bronchoscopy in unresectable tumors. Actuarial survival was 69 months after resection of tracheal adenoid cystic carcinoma and 41 months after bronchoscopy for unresectable adenoid cystic carcinoma. Ten- and 20-year survival rates of resected adenoid cystic carcinoma were 69% and 51% when the airway margins were uninvolved, and 65% and 34% when airway margins were microscopically positive. No patient survived more than 13 years without resection of adenoid cystic carcinoma.

Postintubation Tracheal Stenosis

Background and prevention
The era of widespread mechanical ventilatory support began at the time of the polio epidemic in the late 1940s with the use of tracheal intubation. Within the first decade, the use of tracheostomy for this purpose multiplied, but so also did the incidence of respiratory failure and asphyxiation late after separation from mechanical ventilation and tracheal decannulation. Often, patients would be weaned from ventilation only to develop rapidly progressive airway obstruction either in the hospital or after discharge; many died of acute respiratory failure. Circumferential high-grade tracheal strictures were identified, according to one study in one-fifth of patients undergoing tracheostomy.[23] Careful animal studies showed that high-pressure, poorly compliant tube cuffs that were inflated with air to seal the trachea placed excessive pressure on the tracheal mucosa.[24] The resulting injury advanced from mucosal ulceration overlying the tracheal rings to cartilage erosion, necrosis of cartilage with loss of support, and transmural scar.

The development of treatment and prevention proceeded in parallel. Surgical techniques were devised for segmental resection and reconstruction of the trachea. The transmural nature of these intubation-related strictures demanded excision of the injury: endoscopic therapies with the laser or prosthetic stenting of the lumen failed to restore a reliable lumen, one that would not need repetitive endoscopic intervention; multiple endoscopic procedures often extend the existing injury. In all except the uncommon early injuries that affect only the partial thickness of the tracheal wall, the cartilage skeleton of the trachea is destroyed and requires replacement with normal tracheal wall. The idea of prevention has fundamentally changed the design of endotracheal and tracheostomy tubes with the goal of reducing pressure on the tracheal mucosa: the cuff on these tubes has been replaced with a low-pressure, highly compliant version. While in use for mechanical ventilation, cuff pressures are monitored and maintained below 30 mm Hg, and ideally below 25 mm Hg so that the mucosal perfusion pressure always exceeds cuff pressure. Although these interventions in tube design and intensive care protocol have markedly reduced the incidence, postintubation tracheal stenosis persists even today. Tense overinflation of modern low-pressure cuffs may eventually lead to high pressures and low compliance; a tracheostomy inserted immediately underneath the cricoid may erode the subglottic space; and prolonged dwelling of an endotracheal tube in the glottic aperture may cause a commissural stricture of the vocal cords.

Types of postintubation stenosis

There are at least 4 distinct lesions associated with intubation that are separated here depending on their location within the airway; these lesions differ as well according to type and part of the tube producing the injury. **Fig. 4** shows the injury patterns resulting from intubation. In the differential diagnosis, causes of stricture other than intubation should be considered as listed in **Box 1**.

Glottic stenosis Intubation injury at the glottic level, usually caused by local ischemic effects of prolonged orotracheal tube placement, the selection of an excessively large-caliber tube, or swallowing against the tube, usually develops at the posterior

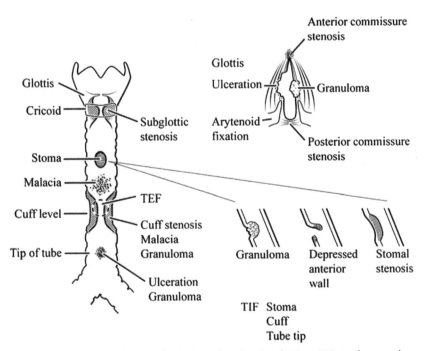

Fig. 4. The various types of tracheal injuries related to intubation. TEF, tracheoesophageal fistula; TIF, tracheoinnominate artery fistula. (*From* Grillo HC. Surgery of the trachea and bronchi. Hamilton, Ontario: BC Decker; 2004. p. 302; with permission.)

Box 1
Causes of benign, nonneoplastic strictures of larynx, trachea, or bronchi

Trauma

    Intubation

    Cicatricial healing of traumatic tear

Infection

    Tuberculosis

    Fungal disease

        Blastomycosis, candidiasis, histoplasmosis, mucormycosis, rhinosporidiosis, coccidiomycosis

    Scleroma

        Klebsiella rhinoscleromatis

    Papillomatosis

Inflammation or autoimmune disease

    Wegener granulomatosis

    Sarcoidosis

    Idiopathic laryngotracheal stenosis

    Relapsing polychondritis

    Amyloidosis

    Tracheopathia osteochondroplastica

---

commissure because this is the area receiving the maximum pressure of the tube. Glottic stenosis is often accompanied by subglottic stenosis for the same reason, and cricoarytenoid joint fixation is a hallmark of severe disease.

Subglottic stenosis Ischemic mucosal changes from prolonged intubation or from intubation with an overly large tube can lead to fibrosis that may significantly narrow the subglottis due to its complete cricoid cartilage ring. Isolated subglottic stenosis can sometimes be managed successfully with serial dilations using ventilating bronchoscopes or balloon dilators,[25] but patients must be assessed for glottic and tracheal involvement to ensure that the entire airway is adequate. Persistent idiopathic strictures are successfully treated with laryngotracheal resection and reconstruction.[26]

Stomal stenosis Healing of a tracheal stoma associated with a large defect of the anterior and lateral wall may produce a triangularly shaped stricture. The anterior projection of the lumen collapses and, although the membranous portion may remain intact, scar contracture of the residual lateral wall results in a tight stenosis. The lumen may accept a dilator, but the expanded lumen achieved by dilatation does not persist.

Cuff stenosis A circumferential stricture at the site of the tube cuff, typically within 3 to 4 cm of the cricoid cartilage but sometimes closer to the carina, is the most common obstructive intubation lesion. Associated with loss of cartilaginous support, the stricture is almost always transmural.

Treatment

The initial management is endoscopic only if airway obstruction is critical. In this situation, dilatation may temporarily enlarge the tracheal diameter; symptoms are expected to recur within weeks, if not earlier. Endoscopic dilatation is described in the section on bronchoscopy. Treated in this manner, tracheal resection is rarely an emergent procedure. Assessment of vocal cord function and integrity of the subglottic larynx should always precede tracheal resection.

Resectable stricture Bronchoscopic measurements of the lengths of trachea and stricture having been obtained, the patient is either intubated with a small (5 to 7 mm) endotracheal tube or, if the obstruction is complete and a tracheostomy exists, across the operative field. The patient is placed supine with elevation of the upper torso and full extension of the neck. A short collar incision with completely mobilized subplatysmal flaps provides exposure to the mid and cervical trachea; an upper midline sternotomy may be added for strictures of the lower trachea or if neck flexion is limited by kyphosis. The thyroid isthmus is divided to reflect the thyroid lobes in cervical strictures. The entire length of the trachea is mobilized in the anterior, avascular plane. The lateral blood vessels must not be disturbed; mobilization of the membranous portion is rarely necessary because the esophagus remains mobile. If not obvious and visible from the outside, the stenotic segment is now marked by introducing an external needle observed with bronchoscopy. Circumferential dissection is carried around the lower end of the stricture keeping the tips of the scissors on the tracheal wall to leave the recurrent laryngeal nerves intact in paratracheal scar. Before the airway is divided, traction sutures are placed around the second or third intact ring cartilage in midlateral position. The airway is divided through stricture, and the quality of the tracheal wall is assessed. Soft scar is excised, while slightly narrowed, but stable trachea is preserved. Only 1 to 1.5 cm of trachea next to the planned anastomosis is circumferentially dissected to maintain its vascular supply. The distal airway is sterilely intubated, and the stricture is excised. With lateral traction sutures in both upper and lower trachea, the neck is flexed to judge tension at the anastomosis. The safe limits of tracheal resection vary with patient age, weight, body habitus, and previous tracheal operations. Usually less than 4 cm of trachea is excised and tension is adequately managed with neck flexion. Young, thin patients may tolerate resection of up to 7 cm of trachea; surgical release maneuvers of larynx and carina[27] lower the amount of tension.

The endotracheal tube is sutured to a small catheter and retracted above the vocal cords. Interrupted, circumferential anastomotic sutures are then placed using 4-0 Vicryl beginning in the midline of the membranous portion and proceeding on either side toward the front. Sutures are spaced 2 to 3 mm apart and 3 to 4 mm deep. Cross-field ventilation is then terminated, the endotracheal tube is returned to the distal trachea, the neck is flexed, and traction sutures are tied first. The anastomotic sutures are tied from the front to the back. The anastomosis is tested for air leaks and covered with thyroid isthmus or strap muscle. If the innominate artery is mobilized during resection, it is protected with a strap muscle flap. A drain is placed. **Fig. 5** depicts the steps of the tracheal anastomosis.

Postintubation strictures involving the subglottic space are assessed before tracheal resection. If the size of the remaining subglottic space is small and the lumen narrowed up to the vocal cords, separate subglottic reconstruction precedes the reconstruction of the trachea. Conversely, subglottic strictures involving the cricoid cartilage may be resected using laryngotracheal reconstruction (**Fig. 6**).

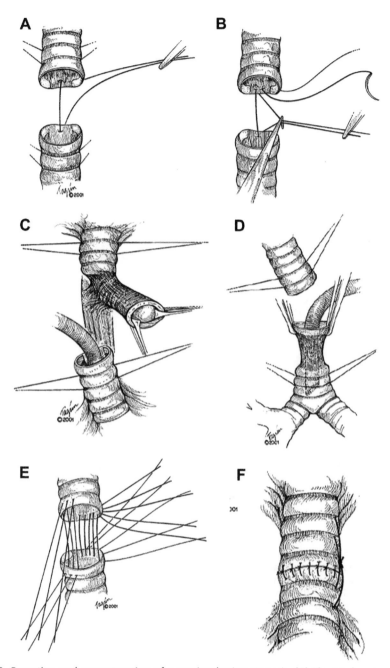

Fig. 5. Resection and reconstruction of a postintubation stenosis. (*A*) The trachea is usually divided below the stricture and the distal airway is intubated. Traction sutures have been placed. (*B*) The trachea may be divided above a low-lying stricture that is then dilated and intubated. The stenosis is excised dissecting immediately on the scar. (*C, D*) The first anastomotic suture is placed in posterior midline inserting additional sutures while retracting the previous ones. (*E, F*) The anastomosis is completed by inserting sutures from posterior to anterior; once the patient's neck has been placed in flexion, the traction sutures are tied first, followed by the anastomotic sutures, now tied from front to back. (*From* Grillo HC. Surgery of the trachea and bronchi. Hamilton, Ontario: BC Decker; 2004. p. 527–38; with permission.)

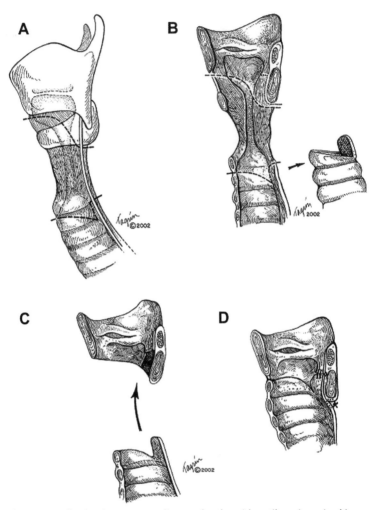

Fig. 6. A laryngotracheal stricture extending to the thyroid cartilage is excised in an oblique manner. The posterior mucosal stricture is excised from the cricoid plate. The distal trachea is tailored in the shape of a prow, leaving a long mucosal flap. The reconstruction covers the cricoid plate with the flap and approximates the cartilaginous trachea to the thyroid cartilage (A–D). (From Grillo HC. Surgery of the trachea and bronchi. Hamilton, Ontario: BC Decker; 2004. p. 559–60; with permission.)

Temporarily or permanently unresectable stricture Surgical reconstruction of postin-tubation tracheal stenosis should be deferred while the patient is mechanically venti-lated, recovering from trauma or medical illness, or is receiving systemic corticosteroids at doses exceeding replacement therapy. Long-segment strictures or subglottic stenosis extending to the vocal cords may be unreconstructable. In the absence of a high subglottic stenosis, the authors prefer the silicone tracheal T-tube[28] (E. Benson Hood Laboratories, Pembroke, MA, or Boston Medical Products, Westborough, MA). The advantages of this type of tracheal stent as compared with self-expanding metal or plastic stents or the Dumon-type stent are the virtual absence of tube-related injury and the ability to suction and clean the trachea. A disadvantage common to all types of tracheal stents is the obligatory bacterial colonization with organisms resistant to multiple antibiotics.

Results

In more than 500 tracheal resections for postintubation stenosis at MGH, 94% of patients achieved a good or satisfactory result and maintain their airway without tracheal tubes. Half of those in whom the first reconstruction failed underwent a second reconstruction.[29]

Tracheomalacia

Tracheomalacia refers to the loss of cartilaginous support of the trachea or major bronchi, resulting in complete or near-complete collapse of the airway lumen during respiration. Malacia may involve isolated segments of the trachea; the cartilages are either destroyed, as in intubation injury, or softened by chronic extrinsic compression, as in congenital vascular malformation or intrathoracic goiters. Acquired diffuse tracheobronchial collapse occurs in the context of chronic obstructive pulmonary disease (COPD) and is believed to represent the chronic inflammatory response of larger airways to tobacco smoke. Tracheal collapse may also present in congenital tracheobronchomegaly, Mounier-Kuhn disease, or in relapsing polychondritis, an autoimmune disease. Intrathoracic collapse occurs during expiration, whereas extra-thoracic malacia results in inspiratory collapse. In patients with emphysema and diffuse malacia, symptoms caused by either disease are difficult to separate. Tracheomalacia in the setting of COPD produces a seal-like bark, a characteristic cough. Asphyxia during obstructive spells may lead to seizures termed laryngeal epilepsy. Recurrent bronchial infections are common and may lead in extreme cases to bronchiectasis.

The diagnosis is made either by MDCT (see section on radiographic evaluation) or by fiberoptic bronchoscopy under light intravenous sedation. Characteristic of the acquired tracheomalacia of COPD is the complete anteroposterior collapse with apposition of cartilage and membranous portion during expiration; inspiration enlarges the lumen. During endoscopic examination, the bronchoscope is placed first into the subglottic space to observe the superior extent of tracheal collapse and is then advanced to either main bronchus to establish the lowest zone of collapse. Thick secretions are invariably found just below the zone of collapse.

Patients with diffuse tracheobronchial malacia are selected for surgical treatment if the severity of malacia exceeds that of small airway disease; this is usually the case when their collapse is complete and extends over the entire trachea. Temporary tracheal stenting may help to assess benefits in individual patients, but is discouraged as long-term therapy because of the complications of endotracheal stenting. Surgical therapy consists of restoring the convex cartilage horseshoe shape by reefing and supporting the membranous wall with polypropylene mesh. The operative technique and the underlying pathophysiologic observations concerning expiratory tracheal collapse were described by Herzog and Nissen in 1954. The operation is conducted through a right thoracotomy, exposing the back wall of the trachea from the thoracic inlet to the lower end of both main bronchi. The trachea is separated from the esophagus for this purpose and the azygous vein is divided. The polypropylene strip is tailored to an approximate width of 2 cm and fixed to the membranous portion with 4 parallel tacking sutures at each level of fixation, with levels separated by about 1 cm. The sutures are clipped with hemostats and tied later, leaving the last row of sutures untied to facilitate placement of the next row. The authors prefer using partial-thickness 4-0 Vicryl sutures; by the time the suture is absorbed, the mesh is already incorporated into the wall. The extent of tracheoplasty and the precise placement of partial-thickness sutures are shown in **Fig. 7**.

Results

The bronchoscopic result is shown in **Fig. 8**. The tracheal and bronchial lumen are inspected before closure of the chest with the bronchoscope to ensure complete correction down to the main bronchial level or, if necessary, to the lobar bronchus. In 14 patients treated with tracheoplasty, mean forced expiratory volume in 1 second rose from 51% predicted to 73%, and peak expiratory flow rate increased from 49% to 70%. During long-term follow-up, 80% of patients had good or excellent results, while 20% had a poor outcome due to collapse of remaining unsplinted bronchi.

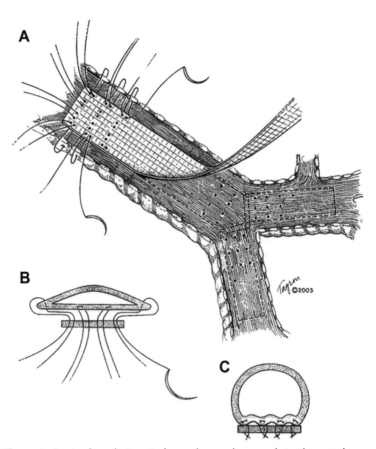

Fig. 7. The posterior tracheoplasty attaches polypropylene mesh to the membranous wall. (*A*) The mesh is carefully tailored and extends to either distal main bronchus. A complete set of 4 sutures is placed each centimeter before tying the last set. (*B*) Proportional spacing of sutures. The lateral sutures grasp the end of the cartilage, all are partial-thickness bites. (*C*) The applied mesh restores the curve of the tracheal cartilage and prevents dynamic collapse during expiration. (*From* Wright CD, Grillo HC, Hammoud ZT, et al. Tracheoplasty for expiratory collapse of central airways. Ann Thorac Surg 2005;80:259–66; with permission.)

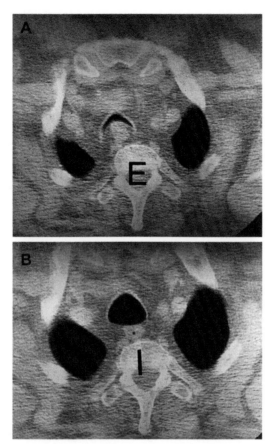

Fig. 8. Multidetector CT study of tracheomalacia during inspiration (*A*) and expiration (*B*). Note near-complete expiratory collapse of the tracheal lumen. (*From* Wright CD, Grillo HC, Hammoud ZT, et al. Tracheoplasty for expiratory collapse of central airways. Ann Thorac Surg 2005;80:259–66; with permission.)

SUMMARY

Careful endoscopic evaluation of acute and chronic airway obstruction identifies a subset of patients with tumors, strictures, or dynamic expiratory collapse who may undergo surgical correction of their obstructive defect. Squamous cell carcinoma and adenoid cystic carcinoma are the most common primary tracheal tumors. These tumors, when of circumscribed length and without metastatic disease, may be resected with resulting long-term survival superior to unresectable disease. Postintubation stenosis is the most common cause of benign tracheal obstruction in developed countries; strictures of limited length are treated with tracheal resection and reconstruction, with satisfactory results in more than 90% of patients. In tracheomalacia related to COPD the surgical correction, tracheoplasty, consists of buttressed reefing of the lax membranous portion to restore the horseshoe shape of the trachea. In experienced hands, tracheal resection has become a routine operation with a predictable outcome.

REFERENCES

1. Brancatisano T, Collett PW, Engel LA. Respiratory movements of the vocal cords. J Appl Physiol 1983;54:1269–76.
2. Salassa JR, Pearson BW, Payne WS. Gross and microscopical blood supply of the trachea. Ann Thorac Surg 1977;24:100–7.
3. Wright CD, Grillo HC, Wain JC, et al. Anastomotic complications after tracheal resection: prognostic factors and management. J Thorac Cardiovasc Surg 2004;128:731–9.
4. Kligerman S, Sharma A. Radiologic evaluation of the trachea. Semin Thorac Cardiovasc Surg 2009;21:246–54.
5. Gaissert HA, Grillo HC, Wright CD, et al. Complication of benign tracheobronchial strictures by self-expanding metal stents. J Thorac Cardiovasc Surg 2003;126:744–7.
6. Food and Drug Administration. FDA public health notification: complications from metallic tracheal stents in patients with benign airway disorders, 2005. Available at: www.fda.gov/MedicalDevices/Safety/AlertsandNotices/PublicHealthNotifications/ucm062115.htm. Accessed July 6, 2010.
7. Mathisen DJ, Grillo HC. Endoscopic relief of malignant airway obstruction. Ann Thorac Surg 1989;48:469–73.
8. Zeitels SM, Akst LM, Burns JA, et al. Office based pulsed KTP-532nm laser treatment of glottal papillomatosis and dysplasia. Ann Otol Rhinol Laryngol 2006;115:679–85.
9. Burns JA, Zeitels SM, Akst LM, et al. 532 nm pulsed potassium-titanyl-phosphate laser treatment of laryngeal papillomatosis under general anesthesia. Laryngoscope 2007;117:1500–4.
10. Burns JA, Har-El G, Shapshay S, et al. Endoscopic laser resection of laryngeal cancer: is it oncologically safe? Position statement from the American Broncho-Esophagological Association. Ann Otol Rhinol Laryngol 2009;118:399–404.
11. Zeitels SM, Burns JA, Lopez-Guerra G, et al. Photoangiolytic laser treatment of early glottic cancer: a new management strategy. Ann Otol Rhinol Laryngol 2008;117(7):1–24, part 2.
12. Ossoff R, Sisson G, Duncavage J, et al. Endoscopic laser arytenoidectomy for the treatment of bilateral vocal cord paralysis. Laryngoscope 1984;94:1293–7.
13. Gaissert HA, Honings J, Grillo HC, et al. Segmental laryngotracheal and tracheal resection for invasive thyroid carcinoma. Ann Thorac Surg 2007;83:1952–9.
14. Gelder CM, Hetzel MR. Primary tracheal tumours: a national survey. Thorax 1993;48:688–92.
15. Gaissert HA, Grillo HC, Shadmehr MB, et al. Uncommon primary tracheal tumors. Ann Thorac Surg 2006;82:268–72.
16. Manninen MP, Pukander JS, Flander MK, et al. Treatment of primary tracheal carcinoma in Finland in 1967–1985. Acta Oncol 1993;32:277–82.
17. Licht PB, Friis S, Pettersson G. Tracheal cancer in Denmark: a nationwide study. Eur J Cardiothorac Surg 2001;19:339–45.
18. Gaissert HA, Grillo HC, Shadmehr MB, et al. Long-term survival after resection of primary adenoid cystic and squamous cell carcinoma of the trachea and carina. Ann Thorac Surg 2004;78:1889–97.
19. Park CM, Goo JM, Lee HJ, et al. Tumors in the tracheobronchial tree: CT and FDG PET features. Radiographics 2009;29:55–71.
20. Regnard JF, Fourquier P, Levasseur P. Results and prognostic factors in resections of primary tracheal tumors: a multicenter retrospective study. The French Society of Cardiovascular Surgery. J Thorac Cardiovasc Surg 1996;111:808–13.

21. Honings J, Gaissert HA, Weinberg AC, et al. Prognostic value of pathologic characteristics and resection margins in tracheal adenoid cystic carcinoma. Eur J Cardiothorac Surg 2010;37:1438–44.
22. Honings J, Gaissert HA, Ruangchira-Urai R, et al. Pathologic characteristics of resected squamous cell carcinoma of the trachea: prognostic factors based on an analysis of 59 cases. Virchows Arch 2009;455:423–9.
23. Head JM. Tracheostomy in the management of respiratory problems. N Engl J Med 1961;264:587–91.
24. Cooper JD, Grillo HC. Experimental production and prevention of injury due to cuffed tracheal tubes. Surg Gynecol Obstet 1969;129:1235–41.
25. Lee KH, Rutter MJ. Role of balloon dilation in the management of adult idiopathic subglottic stenosis. Ann Otol Rhinol Laryngol 2008;117(2):81–4.
26. Grillo HC, Mathisen DJ, Wain JC. Laryngotracheal resection and reconstruction for subglottic stenosis. Ann Thorac Surg 1992;53:54–63.
27. Grillo HC. Surgery of the trachea and bronchi. Hamilton (ON): BC Decker; 2004. (laryngeal release) and 597 (pericardial release) 540–43.
28. Gaissert HA, Grillo HC, Mathisen DJ, et al. Temporary and permanent restoration of airway continuity with the tracheal T-tube. J Thorac Cardiovasc Surg 1994;107: 600–6.
29. Grillo HC, Donahue DM, Mathisen DJ, et al. Postintubation tracheal stenosis. Treatment and results. J Thorac Cardiovasc Surg 1995;109:486–92.

Pediatric Thoracic Problems: Patent Ductus Arteriosus, Vascular Rings, Congenital Tracheal Stenosis, and Pectus Deformities

Hyde M. Russell, MD[a], Carl L. Backer, MD[a,b],*

KEYWORDS

• Patent ductus arteriosus • Trachea • Vascular rings • Pectus
• Chest • Congenital • Pediatric • Surgery

Surgery of the thorax has long been an integral aspect to the care of children, and there are several pediatric thoracic diseases that require surgical attention. In this article the authors focus on 4 of these issues: patent ductus arteriosus, vascular rings, congenital tracheal stenosis, and pectus deformities.

PATENT DUCTUS ARTERIOSUS
Anatomy and Pathophysiology

The ductus arteriosus is a normal fetal structure arising from the left sixth aortic arch connecting the main pulmonary artery and the upper descending thoracic aorta just distal and opposite the origin of the left subclavian artery (**Fig. 1**). The ductus may be bilateral (right and left ductus) or absent. The histologic structure of the ductus arteriosus differs from other arteries with a thick, mucoid filled intima, and a deficiency of medial elastic fibers. It contains disorganized, spiraling smooth muscle cells, which are especially sensitive to prostaglandin-mediated relaxation and PO_2-induced constriction.

Disclosure: The authors have nothing to disclose.
[a] Division of Cardiovascular-Thoracic Surgery, Children's Memorial Hospital, 2300 Children's Plaza, mc 22, Chicago, IL 60614, USA
[b] Northwestern University Feinberg School of Medicine, Chicago, IL 60611, USA
* Corresponding author. Division of Cardiovascular-Thoracic Surgery, Children's Memorial Hospital, 2300 Children's Plaza, mc 22, Chicago, IL 60614.
E-mail address: cbacker@childrensmemorial.org

Surg Clin N Am 90 (2010) 1091–1113
doi:10.1016/j.suc.2010.06.009
0039-6109/10/$ – see front matter © 2010 Elsevier Inc. All rights reserved.

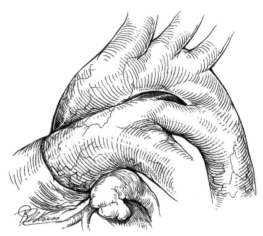

Fig. 1. Patent ductus arteriosus as visualized from a left anterior oblique view. The typical ductus extends from the junction of the main pulmonary artery with the left pulmonary artery to the descending thoracic aorta just distal to the left subclavian artery. (*Reprinted from* Backer CL, Mavroudis C. Patent ductus arteriosus. In: Mavroudis C, Backer CL, editors. Pediatric cardiac surgery, 3rd edition. Philadelphia: Mosby; 2003. p. 224; with permission.)

During fetal development, approximately 60% of the right ventricular blood flow is diverted from the high-resistance pulmonary vascular bed through the patent ductus arteriosus (PDA) into the aorta. Circulating prostaglandins actively maintain ductal patency during fetal life. At birth an elevated arterial PO_2, brought about by breathing, inhibits prostaglandin synthetase, resulting in ductal constriction and eventual fibrosis.[1,2] The fibrosed ductus arteriosus is then called the ligamentum arteriosum.

Natural History

PDA is twice as common among females[3] and occurs in approximately 1 in 1600 term live births.[4] Maternal rubella virus during the first trimester is associated with an increased incidence of PDA.[5] The incidence of PDA in preterm infants is increased in comparison with full-term infants, with an overall incidence of 20% to 30% in the preterm population, rising with earlier gestational age and lower birth weight.[6] The smooth muscle of the infant's pulmonary bed is not sufficiently developed to compensate for the large ductal flow, resulting in pulmonary overcirculation and congestive heart failure. In addition, retrograde blood flow from the descending aorta into the pulmonary circulation through the ductus during diastole leads to decreased systemic flow and a predisposition to end-organ ischemia, including necrotizing enterocolitis, renal insufficiency, abnormal cerebral blood flow, and chronic lung disease.

In term infants and older children, a small PDA may be hemodynamically insignificant and detected only by echocardiography. A large nonrestrictive ductus with no other congenital cardiac defects produces a large left-to-right shunt with left atrial dilation, left ventricular volume overload, and progressive congestive heart failure. Left untreated, a large PDA may lead to pulmonary arteriolar hypertension with the eventual development of a right-to-left shunt and Eisenmenger physiology. Significant elevation in pulmonary vascular resistance may develop as early as 6 months of life, resulting in suprasystemic pulmonary artery pressures. Other complications, reported less frequently today than in historical series, include infective endocarditis,[2] ductal aneurysm,[7] aortic aneurysm, pulmonary artery aneurysm, and aortic dissection.

In the current era, the risk of developing congestive heart failure and/or pulmonary hypertension with a moderate or large ductus along with the (low) risk of bacterial endocarditis for even a small ductus are indications for surgical intervention in nearly all patients with an isolated (clinically audible) PDA. The management of the "silent" PDA detected only by echocardiogram and estimated to be present in 0.5% of the population remains controversial.

Clinical Features and Diagnosis

Symptoms and physical findings depend on the age of the patient and the size of the ductus, as well as the pulmonary vascular resistance and associated intracardiac defects. Infants with a large PDA develop heart failure from pulmonary overcirculation in the first weeks of life manifested by tachypnea, tachycardia, and poor feeding. Physical findings include an overactive precordium, wide pulse pressure, and an enlarged liver. Preterm infants with a large ductus will frequently have respiratory distress and require intubation and ventilation.

The shunt through a moderate-sized PDA increases significantly over the first few months of life as the pulmonary vascular resistance falls. These children tend to have failure to thrive, recurrent upper respiratory tract infections, and fatigue with exertion. In an older child with a small restrictive ductus the diagnosis is usually made at the time of a child's preschool physical examination, with a typical continuous "machinery" murmur heard in the left second intercostal space.

Radiographic findings are proportional to the degree of left-to-right shunting; a large ductus results in enlargement of the left atrium and left ventricle, increased pulmonary vascular markings, and interstitial pulmonary edema. Electrocardiographic changes indicative of left ventricular hypertrophy and left atrial enlargement are often present. Transthoracic echocardiography, the diagnostic method of choice, can accurately identify the ductal anatomy and characterize shunt flow.[8] Cardiac catheterization is necessary only when echocardiogram findings suggest severe pulmonary hypertension or if the patient is a candidate for transcatheter closure. Patients with fixed pulmonary hypertension will have systemic desaturation and can exhibit differential cyanosis, with a pink face and right hand, and cyanosis of the feet. These patients are not candidates for ductal closure because of the high risk of right ventricular failure, and must be considered candidates for lung transplantation and simultaneous PDA closure.[9]

Treatment

There are many different treatment strategies now available for the child with a PDA. These approaches include pharmacologic therapy for premature infants (indomethacin), closure in the catheterization laboratory (coils, occluder devices), video-assisted thoracoscopic clip closure, and thoracotomy with ligation or division and oversewing.

Medical Management

Indomethacin (an inhibitor of prostaglandin synthetase) has been applied clinically since 1976 to constrict the ductus and facilitate closure in premature infants.[10] In full-term infants, indomethacin therapy is rarely successful. A schedule of 3 doses of 0.1 to 0.2 mg/kg administered intravenously every 12 to 24 hours has been widely used. The efficacy of indomethacin as compared with simple medical therapy for a PDA (ventilator support, fluid restriction, and diuretics) in premature infants is well documented. Gersony and colleagues[11] demonstrated a 79% incidence of duct closure with indomethacin in premature infants, and this has become the standard for initial management of preterm infants with a significant ductus. If indomethacin is contraindicated (due to sepsis, coagulation abnormalities, or renal insufficiency) or if closure is not obtained following 3 courses of indomethacin, conversion to a surgical closure strategy is indicated.

Early surgical closure of PDA in preterm infants carries a very low operative morbidity and mortality.[12] Compared with medical management (excluding indomethacin therapy), a randomized trial demonstrated that surgical ligation reduces the need for mechanical ventilation and oxygen therapy, shortens hospital stay, and decreases complications such as necrotizing enterocolitis.[13] Many centers, including the authors', now perform PDA ligation in the neonatal intensive care unit at the bedside, avoiding the potential complications in transporting these critically ill infants. This strategy allows for uninterrupted ventilation with the neonatal ventilator and maintenance of normothermia.

Surgical Technique

The infant is placed in the right lateral decubitus position. Blood pressure and pulse oximetry monitors are placed on the right hand and a lower extremity to monitor perfusion. The chest is entered through a muscle-sparing third or fourth interspace posterolateral thoracotomy, and the lung is retracted anteriorly. The mediastinal pleura is opened longitudinally (**Fig. 2**). Misinterpretation of the anatomic details can lead to inadvertent ligation of the descending aorta or left pulmonary artery, therefore all structures must be carefully identified.[14,15] Most mistakes occur because the large ductus is misinterpreted as being the actual arch of the aorta. Extensive dissection of the ductus in preterm infants is inadvisable; tissues may be friable and life-threatening hemorrhage may ensue. The recurrent laryngeal nerve should be identified, and steps taken to preserve it. The ductus is encircled and ligated with a single strand of 2-0 silk (4-0 silk in small premature infants), is clipped with a metal hemoclip, or both (**Fig. 3**). Care must be taken with both techniques not to cut through the very soft neonatal ductal tissue. While it is acceptable to simply ligate or hemoclip the PDA in preterm infants, all other patients should have double or triple ligation or division and oversewing to minimize the risk of incomplete closure or recanalization. In addition to the silk ligature, a purse-string suture of 5-0 polypropylene, placed superficially in the adventitia, is used to close the pulmonary end of the ductus.[16,17]

In older children and adults the authors recommend division and oversewing because of the incidence of incomplete closure, estimated at 0.2% to 6% in recent series with ligation alone.[18–20] In this technique, the ductus arteriosus is dissected free with enough length to place Potts ductus clamps and have adequate ductal stumps to oversew.[16] After dissection, the ductus is clamped with 2 Potts vascular clamps, divided, and the cuff of ductus in each clamp is oversewn with 2 rows of continuous fine polypropylene suture (**Fig. 4**). The clamp on the pulmonary side is removed first, as it is less likely to bleed.

Hemodynamic changes associated with closure of the ductus include a significant increase in systolic and particularly diastolic blood pressure. The mediastinal pleura are left open in premature infants, as it is usually too friable to close; in all other patients it is routinely closed. The pneumothorax is evacuated with a small suction catheter following rib reapproximation. Although the authors previously placed a chest tube in these patients for 24 hours, Miles and colleagues[21] have shown that this is not necessary, and the authors now do not leave a chest tube unless there is an obvious air leak from the lung.

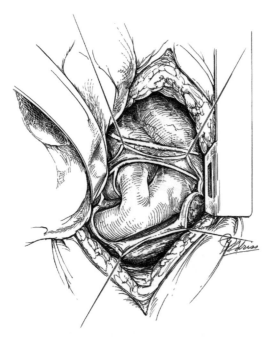

Fig. 2. Operative exposure of a patent ductus arteriosus (PDA) through a left thoracotomy. The mediastinal pleura is opened and reflected anteriorly and posteriorly. The vagus and recurrent laryngeal nerves are identified and preserved by retracting them medially. (*Reprinted from* Backer CL, Mavroudis C. Patent ductus arteriosus. In: Mavroudis C, Backer CL, editors. Pediatric cardiac surgery, 3rd edition. Philadelphia: Mosby; 2003. p. 227; with permission.)

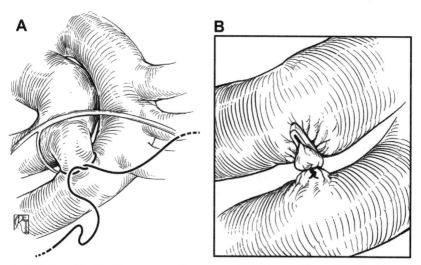

Fig. 3. Techniques for ligation, multiple ligation, and ligation and hemoclip of patent ductus arteriosus. Exposure is via a left muscle-sparing thoracotomy. (*A*) Ligation with a single 2-0 silk ligature. (*B*) Ligation with a 2-0 silk and placement of a hemoclip. (*Reprinted from* Backer CL, Mavroudis C. Patent ductus arteriosus. In: Mavroudis C, Backer CL, editors. Pediatric cardiac surgery, 3rd edition. Philadelphia: Mosby; 2003. p. 227; with permission.)

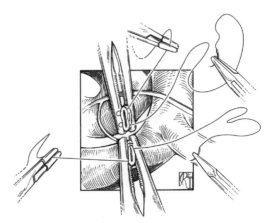

Fig. 4. Technique of ductal division and oversewing. The aortic and pulmonary stumps of the ductus are oversewn with continuous double rows of 5-0 polypropylene sutures, first layer as a horizontal mattress suture, second layer as a simple over-and-over suture. (*Reprinted from* Backer CL, Mavroudis C. Patent ductus arteriosus. In: Mavroudis C, Backer CL, editors. Pediatric cardiac surgery, 3rd edition. Philadelphia: Mosby; 2003. p. 229; with permission.)

Small infants are recovered and remain in the neonatal intensive care unit following the bedside procedure. Older children go to the regular recovery room and then to the ward. Most patients are discharged in 24 to 36 hours. Using this technique at Children's Memorial Hospital between 1947 and 1993, 1108 patients underwent division and oversewing of a PDA with no mortality and minimal morbidity, and no recurrence.[22] There was a 1.2% incidence of transient recurrent laryngeal nerve injury and a 0.3% incidence of reoperation for bleeding (none in the past 25 years).

In adult patients the PDA may be short, thin-walled, and have calcific changes in the ductus, which makes "routine" division or ligation hazardous. In these circumstances, the PDA should be approached through a median sternotomy with the support of cardiopulmonary bypass.[23]

Alternative Closure Strategies

Video-Assisted Thoracoscopic Surgery (VATS) interruption and catheter-based endovascular coiling represent 2 alternative strategies to close a PDA. VATS can be performed using 3-, 4-, or 5-mm port sites for instrumentation. Division of the intercostal muscles, spreading of the ribs, and stretching of the paraspinal muscles are reduced, thereby decreasing chest wall trauma, pain, and recovery time.[24] Percutaneous catheter-based treatment is possible in the older infant and child with a variety of endovascular closure devices, with acceptable results. The authors' current institutional policy is to recommend coil occlusion of small to moderate size (<5 mm) PDAs and a muscle-sparing thoracotomy with division and oversewing of moderate to large PDAs. Enthusiasm for this strategy is based on the very low risk, low cost, and ease of coil placement for smaller PDAs, and the essential guarantee of no residual shunt, no mortality, and minimal morbidity with the division and oversewing technique in more than 1000 patients in the authors' institution.[25]

VASCULAR RINGS

The term "vascular ring" is used to describe vascular anomalies that result from abnormal development of the aortic arch complex and cause compression of the trachea, esophagus, or both. Most children with vascular rings present with symptoms in the first few months of life and require surgery within the first year of life.[25] Some of these anomalies are anatomically complete rings, or true vascular rings (double aortic arch and right arch/left ligament); others are anatomically incomplete, or partial vascular rings (innominate artery compression and pulmonary sling), but present similar symptoms because of the tracheoesophageal compression.

Double Aortic Arch

If the right and left fourth arches both persist, a double aortic arch is formed (**Fig. 5**). Two arches arise from the ascending aorta and pass on both sides of the trachea and esophagus, joining the descending aorta, producing a true ring. The right (posterior) arch gives origin to the right carotid and subclavian arteries. The left carotid and subclavian arteries arise from the usually smaller left (anterior) arch. In 70% of these infants, the right-sided arch is dominant, in 20% the left arch is dominant, and in 5% the arches are equal in size. The trachea and esophagus are encircled and compressed by the two arches.

Right Aortic Arch

If the left fourth arch involutes, a right aortic arch system is created (see **Fig. 5**). The apex of the aortic arch in these patients is to the right of the trachea. Depending on the exact site(s) of interruption of the left arch and the branching pattern to the left

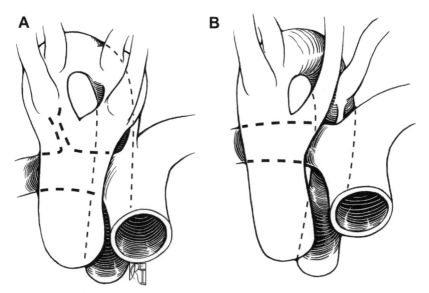

Fig. 5. Diagram of the embryonic aortic arches. Six pairs of aortic arches originally develop between the dorsal and ventral aorta. The first, second, and fifth arches regress. Preservation or deletion of different segments of the rudimentary arches results in either a double aortic arch, a right aortic arch, or the "normal" left aortic arch (A, B). (*Reprinted from* Backer CL, Mavroudis C. Patent ductus arteriosus. In: Mavroudis C, Backer CL, editors. Pediatric cardiac surgery, 3rd edition. Philadelphia: Mosby; 2003. p. 235; with permission.)

subclavian artery, left carotid artery, and ductus arteriosus, different configurations of right aortic arch are possible (**Fig. 6**). The 2 common variations are retroesophageal left subclavian artery (65%) and mirror-image branching (35%).[26] The right aortic arch with a retroesophageal left subclavian artery results from persistence of the right fourth arch and deletion of the left arch between the left carotid and subclavian arteries. The subclavian artery originates from the descending aorta and courses to the left behind the esophagus. The ligamentum nearly always extends from the descending aorta to the left pulmonary artery, completing the vascular ring (**Fig. 6**A). A right aortic arch with mirror-image branching and left ligamentum arteriosum results from persistence of the right fourth aortic arch and disappearance of the left arch between the subclavian artery and the dorsal descending aorta. When the

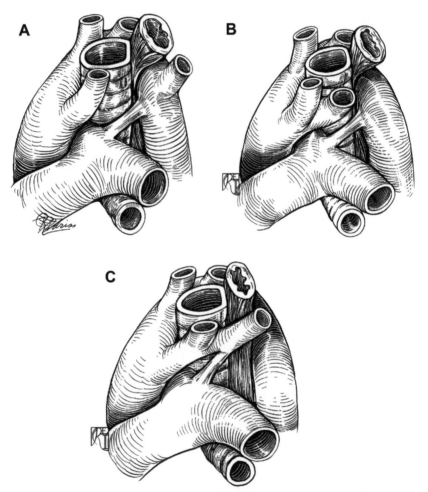

Fig. 6. Right aortic arch types. (*A*) Retroesophageal left subclavian artery, ligamentum to descending aorta. (*B*) Mirror-image branching, ligamentum to descending aorta. (*C*) Mirror-image branching, ligamentum to left innominate artery. (*Reprinted from* Backer CL, Mavroudis C. Patent ductus arteriosus. In: Mavroudis C, Backer CL, editors. Pediatric cardiac surgery, 3rd edition. Philadelphia: Mosby; 2003. p. 236; with permission.)

ligamentum originates from the descending aorta, a complete vascular ring is formed
(**Fig. 6**B). If the ligamentum originates from the innominate artery, which is more
common in this group, a vascular ring is not formed and the child is asymptomatic
(**Fig. 6**C).

Pulmonary Artery Sling

The embryonic origin of pulmonary artery sling occurs when the developing left lung
captures its arterial supply from derivatives of the right sixth arch through capillaries
caudal rather than cephalad to the developing tracheobronchial tree.[27] The left pulmonary artery originates from the right pulmonary artery instead of the main pulmonary
artery. The left pulmonary artery passes around the right main bronchus and courses
between the trachea and esophagus, forming a "sling" that compresses the tracheobronchial tree (**Fig. 7**). The airway may also be compromised by associated complete
cartilage tracheal rings, the so-called ring-sling complex, where the membranous
portion of the trachea is absent and the tracheal cartilages are circumferential (see
Fig. 7).[28]

Innominate Artery Compression

Innominate artery compression syndrome results from anterior compression of the
trachea by the innominate artery. Why an innominate artery, which normally crosses
in front of the trachea, should compress the trachea in some cases and not others
is not well understood. The innominate artery appears to originate somewhat more
posteriorly and leftward on the aortic arch than usual. As the artery courses to the
right, upward, and posterior to reach the right thoracic outlet, it compresses the
trachea anteriorly (**Fig. 8**).[29]

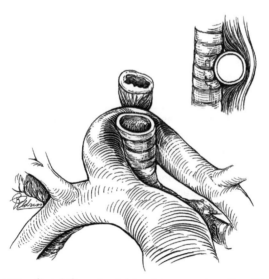

Fig. 7. Pulmonary artery sling. left; main, right pulmonary artery. (*Inset*) Left lateral view of
anterior compression of the esophagus of anterior trachea. (*Reprinted from* Backer CL,
Mavroudis C. Patent ductus arteriosus. In: Mavroudis C, Backer CL, editors. Pediatric cardiac
surgery, 3rd edition. Philadelphia: Mosby; 2003. p. 237; with permission.)

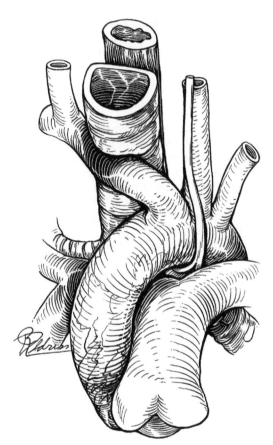

Fig. 8. Innominate artery compression of anterior trachea. (*Reprinted from* Backer CL, Mavroudis C. Patent ductus arteriosus. In: Mavroudis C, Backer CL, editors. Pediatric cardiac surgery, 3rd edition. Philadelphia: Mosby; 2003. p. 237; with permission.)

Clinical Presentation and Diagnosis

Most children with vascular rings present with symptoms within the first several weeks to months of life. Double aortic arch and pulmonary sling are particularly symptomatic and present earlier than other lesions. The symptoms typically include some combination of the following: respiratory distress, stridor, the classic "seal bark" cough, apnea, dysphagia, and recurrent respiratory tract infections. Infants may hold their head hyperextended to splint the trachea and lessen the obstruction, improving their breathing. As infants progress from liquid formula to solid food, symptoms of dysphagia may become more evident. Some older children will present only with symptoms of dysphagia or slow feeding where they tend to be the last child to leave the table because they have to chew their food carefully as a learned procedure. The diagnosis of vascular rings requires a high index of suspicion because of the relative infrequency of this diagnosis compared with other conditions that cause respiratory distress in children such as asthma, reflux, and upper respiratory tract infection. Symptoms appear earlier and tend to be more severe in cases with a double aortic arch. Children with innominate artery compression syndrome present with symptoms of tracheal compression, and nearly one-half have had apneic episodes. It is important in these infants to rule out other causes of apneic spells by including a complete neurologic evaluation, investigation for gastroesophageal reflux, and sleep studies. Physical examination may reveal stridor, wheezing, tachypnea, a brassy cough, or noisy breathing. If the obstruction is severe there may be obvious subcostal retractions, and nasal flaring.

The diagnosis of a vascular ring starts with the plain chest radiograph. There are a myriad of other diagnostic procedures that may be employed, including barium esophagogram, bronchoscopy, tracheograms, computed tomography (CT), magnetic resonance imaging, echocardiography, and cardiac catheterization. In the authors' practice a CT-angiogram is the single best test when the lesion is suspected.[30] Because of the speed of modern CT scanners, the test generally does not require general anesthesia. It can confirm or refute the diagnosis in a noninvasive manner and provides a very accurate road map of the great vessels for the surgeon. Furthermore, it aids surgical planning by demonstrating the presence of a Kommerell diverticulum, revealing dominance of the right or left arch in the case of a double arch, and the anatomy of a pulmonary artery sling.

Surgical Management

An operation is indicated in all symptomatic patients who have a vascular ring.[31] Initiation of early and appropriate surgical treatment is important to avoid serious complications that may arise after hypoxic or apneic spells. Delayed treatment may result in either sudden death or further tracheobronchial damage. All patients brought to the operating room with a vascular ring should undergo bronchoscopy to define the level and extent of tracheal narrowing and evaluate for complete tracheal rings or other unexpected pathology. The surgical approach varies depending on the specific vascular ring diagnosed. A left posterolateral thoracotomy provides excellent exposure in almost all cases of the true vascular rings (ie, double aortic arch and right aortic arch with left ligamentum). The authors use a right thoracotomy for the innominate artery compression syndrome and other rare vascular rings,[32] and a median sternotomy for pulmonary artery sling with or without complete tracheal rings.

Double aortic arch

Nearly all of these patients are best approached through a left thoracotomy. The exception is the patient with a dominant left arch, where the approach is best with a right thoracotomy. The left thoracotomy can be performed with a muscle-sparing technique, elevating the serratus and latissimus muscles and entering the thorax through the fourth intercostal space. The mediastinal pleura are widely opened. Careful dissection in the posterior mediastinum should be performed to clearly delineate the anatomic configuration of the vascular ring. In particular, the left subclavian artery, ligamentum arteriosum, and descending aorta should be identified (**Fig. 9**A). The left (anterior) arch typically is the smaller of the 2 arches, and it may be atretic where it inserts into the descending aorta. The vascular ring caused by the double aortic arch is released by dividing the lesser of the 2 arches, usually at the posterior insertion site into the descending aorta. The lesser arch is divided between clamps at a site selected to preserve brachiocephalic blood flow (**Fig. 9**B). Pulse oximetry tracings from both upper extremities as well as bilateral carotid pulsations are confirmed after clamping and before division. The ring is divided and the stumps oversewn with a double layer of running polypropylene suture. In addition, the ligamentum arteriosum is always ligated and divided, and careful dissection performed around the esophagus and the trachea to lyse any residual adhesive bands. The recurrent laryngeal nerve and

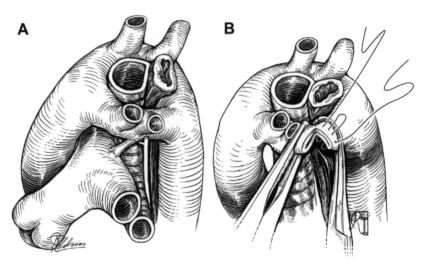

Fig. 9. Double aortic arch division. (*A*) Double aortic arch, right arch dominant. (*B*) Dividing left aortic arch. (*Reprinted from* Backer CL, Mavroudis C. Patent ductus arteriosus. In: Mavroudis C, Backer CL, editors. Pediatric cardiac surgery, 3rd edition. Philadelphia: Mosby; 2003. p. 243; with permission.)

phrenic nerve are identified and protected throughout the case. Of importance, the mediastinal pleura are left widely open to decrease the chance of recurrent stenosis in the area of ring division.

Right aortic arch with left ligamentum

For the patient with a right aortic arch and a left ligamentum, the same left thoracotomy muscle-sparing approach is used. After careful dissection and identification of the configuration of the aortic arch, the ligamentum arteriosum is identified. The ligamentum is either doubly ligated and divided or doubly clamped and divided with the 2 stumps oversewn (**Fig. 10**). Any adhesive bands are lysed and the recurrent laryngeal nerve and phrenic nerve are carefully identified and protected. Patients with a right aortic arch and a left ligamentum may have a Kommerell diverticulum at the origin of the left subclavian artery from the descending aorta.[33] This diverticulum may enlarge to proportions that can independently compress the esophagus or trachea, or even rupture.[34] If the diverticulum or aneurysmal dilatation is 1.5 to 2.0 times the diameter of the left subclavian artery, it should be resected and the left subclavian artery transferred to the left carotid artery to prevent its independent compression of the trachea and esophagus (**Fig. 11**).[35]

Innominate artery compression syndrome

The management of compression of the trachea by the innominate artery has classically been with suspension of the innominate artery to the posterior aspect of the sternum.[36] The authors' approach for these patients is via a small right submammary anterolateral thoracotomy (**Fig. 12**). The right lobe of the thymus is excised, taking care not to injure the right phrenic nerve. No dissection is performed between the innominate artery and the trachea so as not to release the anterior traction on the trachea following suspension. The innominate artery is suspended with pledget-supported sutures to the posterior periosteum of the sternum to lift the innominate artery away from the trachea, simultaneously pulling open the anterior

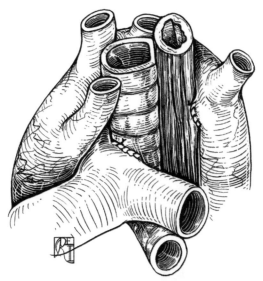

Fig. 10. Right aortic arch division and oversewing of ligamentum arteriosum. (*Reprinted from* Backer CL, Mavroudis C. Patent ductus arteriosus. In: Mavroudis C, Backer CL, editors. Pediatric cardiac surgery, 3rd edition. Philadelphia: Mosby; 2003. p. 244; with permission.)

tracheal wall. Typically, 3 separate mattress sutures are used. The first is on the anterior surface of the aortic arch in line with the origin of the innominate artery, the second at the junction between the innominate artery and the aorta, and the third 0.5 cm distal to the origin of the innominate artery. A right upper extremity arterial line or pulse oximetry tracing confirms patency of the innominate artery during this manipulation. Bronchoscopy is then performed after the suspension to confirm relief of the tracheal compression.

Pulmonary artery sling
The first pulmonary artery sling repair was performed by Willis Potts at Children's Memorial Hospital in 1953.[37] Through a right thoracotomy he doubly clamped and transected the left pulmonary artery, translocated it anterior to the trachea, and then reimplanted it into the original division site on the right pulmonary artery. The procedure has evolved since that first operation. The authors currently advocate an approach with median sternotomy and the use of extracorporeal circulation.[38,39] This approach allows accurate transection of the left pulmonary artery with implantation into the main pulmonary artery anterior to the trachea (**Fig. 13**). The operation can be performed without respiratory compromise (patient is on cardiopulmonary bypass), and enough time and care can be taken to ensure patency of the left pulmonary artery.

Tracheal stenosis
The surgical treatment of complete tracheal rings has undergone an evolution at Children's Memorial Hospital from the first pericardial patch procedure performed in 1982, to the tracheal autograft technique, to the slide tracheoplasty.[40–44] The current procedures of choice for infants with congenital tracheal stenosis are resection with end-to-end anastomosis for short-segment stenosis (up to 6 rings) and the slide tracheoplasty for long-segment stenosis. The slide tracheoplasty is performed through a median

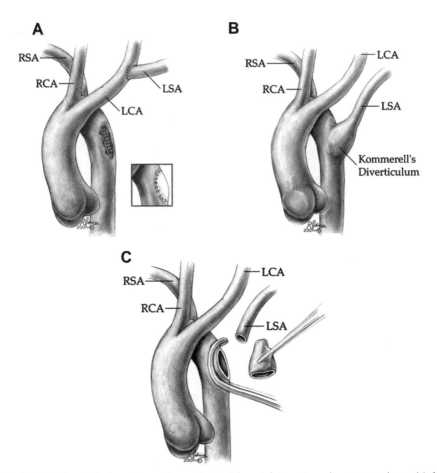

Fig. 11. (*A*) The typical anatomy of a patient with a right aortic arch, retroesophageal left subclavian artery, and large Kommerell diverticulum. The Kommerell diverticulum is an embryologic remnant of the left fourth aortic arch. (*B*) Resection of a Kommerell diverticulum through a left thoracotomy. There is a vascular clamp partially occluding the descending thoracic aorta at the origin of the Kommerell diverticulum. The Kommerell diverticulum has been completely resected. The clamp on the distal left subclavian artery is not illustrated. (*C*). The completed repair. The orifice where the Kommerell diverticulum was resected is usually closed primarily or, as shown in the inset, the orifice can be patched with polytetrafluoroethylene if necessary. The left subclavian artery has been implanted into the side of the left common carotid artery with fine running polypropylene suture. LCA/RCA, left/right carotid artery; LSA/RSA, left/right subclavian artery. (*From* Backer CL, Hillman N, Mavroudis C, et al. Resection of Kommerell diverticulum and left subclavian artery: transfer for recurrent symptoms after vascular ring division. Eur J Cardiothorac Surg 2002;22:44; with permission.)

sternotomy with extracorporeal circulation. The authors use a collar incision in the neck like a "T" (at the top of the sternotomy incision) to adequately visualize the cervical portion of the trachea. If a pulmonary artery sling or cardiac anomaly is present, those are repaired first. After initiating cardiopulmonary bypass with an aortic and single atrial venous cannula, the trachea is divided in the midportion of the

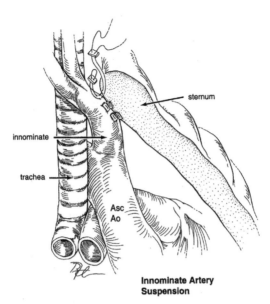

**Innominate Artery
Suspension**

Fig. 12. Innominate artery suspension. Exposure is through a right submammary thoracotomy. Fixing the adventitia of the innominate artery to the posterior table of the sternum with pledgeted sutures pulls the innominate artery anteriorly and actively pulls the tracheal wall forward and opens it. Asc. Ao, ascending aorta. (*Reprinted from* Backer CL, Mavroudis C. Surgical approach to vascular rings. In: Karp R, Laks H, Wechsler AS, editors. Advances in cardiac surgery, vol. 9. St Louis (MO): Mosby-Year Book; 1997. p. 49; with permission.)

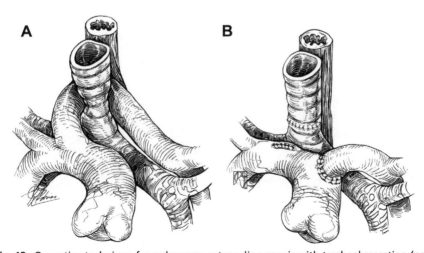

Fig. 13. Operative technique for pulmonary artery sling repair with tracheal resection (performed with cardiopulmonary bypass). (*A*) Left pulmonary artery encircles and compresses distal area of trachea and right main stem bronchus. (*B*) Relationship of left pulmonary artery to trachea and esophagus. (*Reprinted from* Backer CL, Mavroudis C. Patent ductus arteriosus. In: Mavroudis C, Backer CL, editors. Pediatric cardiac surgery, 3rd edition. Philadelphia: Mosby; 2003. p. 246; with permission.)

tracheal stenosis. This location is determined either by external visual inspection or fiberoptic bronchoscopy. The inferior portion of the trachea is incised anteriorly and the superior portion of the trachea is incised posteriorly. The corners of the tracheal openings are trimmed. An anastomosis is performed with running 5-0 or 6-0 polydioxanone suture starting at the superior aspect and finishing by the carina (**Fig 14**). The patient then undergoes bronchoscopy to aspirate secretions and to ensure that the stenosis has been relieved. The repair is stented with an endotracheal tube for 3 to 5 days, and the child is kept on a ventilator. The authors use diluted nebulized ciprodex every 6 to 8 hours to reduce granulation tissue. Follow-up bronchoscopy is performed to remove granulation tissue, clear secretions, and identify residual stenosis. The child is then weaned from the ventilator and extubated.

Results

One hundred and thirty-nine patients have had repair of a double aortic arch at Children's Memorial Hospital with no operative mortality from repair of an isolated double aortic arch since 1952. Two patients required reoperation for persistent symptoms arising from scar tissue at the divided posterior left arch. One hundred and forty patients at Children's Memorial Hospital have had division of the ligamentum for a diagnosis of right aortic arch, retroesophageal left subclavian artery, and left ligamentum. There has been no operative mortality since 1959. No patient in these series has required a reoperation. Thirty-seven patients underwent resection of a Kommerell diverticulum, 19 of whom required transfer of the left subclavian artery to the left carotid artery. Nearly all patients were extubated in the operating room. The patients are monitored overnight in the cardiac intensive care unit, and discharged home on the second or third postoperative day. In most cases, it takes weeks to months for the barky cough to completely disappear, although it is nearly always significantly improved immediately postoperatively.

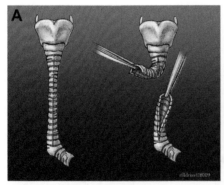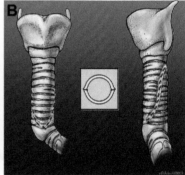

Fig. 14. Slide tracheoplasty; absent right lung. (*A*) The patient has been placed on cardiopulmonary bypass with mild hypothermia to 32°C. The trachea is transected in the midportion of the tracheal stenosis. This site is determined by either external examination or by internal bronchoscopic findings. The inferior portion of the trachea is incised anteriorly and the superior portion of the trachea is incised posteriorly. (*B*) The ends of the trachea are beveled as shown in the small inset. The anastomosis is performed with running 6-0 polydioxanone suture. The suture line is started superiorly (parachute technique) and finished inferiorly just above the carina. (*Reprinted from* Backer CL, Kelle AM, Mavroudis C, et al. Tracheal reconstruction in children with unilateral lung agenesis or severe hypoplasia. Ann Thorac Surg 2009;88:428; with permission.)

Eighty-seven patients have had innominate arteriopexy at Children's Memorial Hospital. There have been no operative mortalities for isolated innominate artery suspension. Two patients have required reoperation for resuspension.

Forty patients have undergone repair of pulmonary artery sling at the authors' institution between 1953 and 2008 at a median age of 4 months. There were no operative mortalities and 4 late deaths from respiratory complications. All patients operated on in the current era with the use of cardiopulmonary bypass have patent left pulmonary arteries documented by nuclear scanning.

The results of repair of tracheal stenosis at Children's Memorial Hospital encompass 3 different operative techniques in 75 patients over a 27-year time period. Twenty-five patients (33%) had an associated pulmonary sling, and 17 patients (23%) had an intracardiac abnormality. There were 7 early deaths (9%) and 5 late deaths (7%). Seven patients required a tracheostomy.

CHEST WALL DEFORMITIES

Pectus excavatum and carinatum represent 2 of the most common pediatric abnormalities of the chest wall. The deformity has been recognized for many years, yet the indications for surgery, ideal timing of operation, and method of repair remain controversial. A brief overview of the issues is presented.

Clinical Presentation

Patients with pectus excavatum may suffer from decreased exercise tolerance, exercise-induced asthma, and pain whereas patients with pectus carinatum typically complain of pain and frequent injuries to their elevated sternum during sporting activities. Both subsets of patients may have body image issues, which drive the patients or their parents to seek medical attention.

Physical examination reveals the typical depressed or protruded chest. The maximal distance of the deformity can be measured grossly in the examining room by placing a level marker across the chest and measuring down to the nadir of the excavatum chest wall or up to the peak of the carinatum. The authors obtain posteroanterior and lateral plain chest radiographs and noncontrast CT scans in all patients. The Haller index is obtained by measuring the lateral width of the chest at the point of the excavatum and dividing by the anteroposterior distance between the sternum and the anterior spine, with a value of 3.25 considered severe in the setting of pectus excavatum.[45] A similar index does not exist for pectus carinatum. Echocardiography reveals compression of right-sided cardiac structures in severe cases of pectus excavatum. The authors' practice is to offer operation to patients with a Haller index greater than 3.25 and those with evidence of cardiorespiratory symptoms and echocardiographic abnormalities.

Surgical Technique

The preferred technique is a modification of the Ravitch operation, first described in 1949.[46] Patients are offered epidural catheters for postoperative analgesia at the discretion of the anesthesiologist. A limited vertical midline incision is centered over the defect. Skin flaps are raised with electrocautery to the midclavicular line bilaterally. The pectoralis muscle is divided in the midline reflected laterally and the rectus muscle mobilized inferiorly, exposing the inferior cartilages. A subperichondrial resection of all deformed cartilages (usually cartilages 3–6 or 3–7) is then performed with a Freer elevator. The xyphoid is freed from the rectus attachments. The intercostal muscle bundles and perichondrial sheaths are dissected free of the sternum with electrocautery (**Fig 15**). For pectus excavatum deformities, an anterior sternal osteotomy is performed with an osteotome just inferior to the last normal costal cartilage, leaving the posterior cortex intact. The posterior table is fractured and angulated anteriorly, without displacement, to maintain an adequate blood supply. Two heavy Ticron (Davis & Geck, Manati, PR) sutures are placed to close the wedge after the sternum has been elevated to the desired position (**Fig. 16**A). A stainless steel substernal bar (V. Mueller Co, Allegiance Healthcare Corp, Deerfield, IL) is used in all cases of pectus excavatum and is placed at the fourth or fifth intercostal space. The bar extends from the right anterior axillary line to the left anterior axillary line anterior to the ribs and posterior to the sternum (**Fig. 16**B). The ends are bent to conform to the contour of the ribs and are transfixed with absorbable sutures (0 Maxon [Davis & Geck]) to the rib and the sternum bilaterally. In pectus carinatum deformities a bar is not routinely used, and a posterior sternal osteotomy is performed. After resection of a triangular wedge of the sternum, the sternum is fractured and angulated posteriorly without displacement to the desired position. Reattachment of the perichondrial sheaths to the sternal edges (see **Fig 16**B), followed by reapproximation of the rectus and pectoralis muscles and skin flaps complete the operation (**Fig 17**). Pliable, closed suction

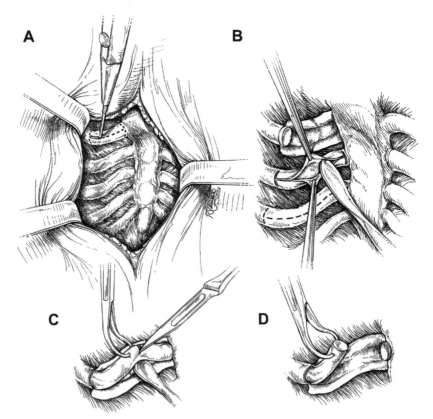

Fig. 15. (*A–D*) The perichondrial sheaths and intercostals muscle bundles are dissected free of the sternum bilaterally. (*Reprinted from* Willekes CL, Backer CL, Mavroudis C. A 26-year review of pectus deformity repairs, including simultaneous intracardiac repair. Ann Thorac Surg 1999;67:512; with permission.)

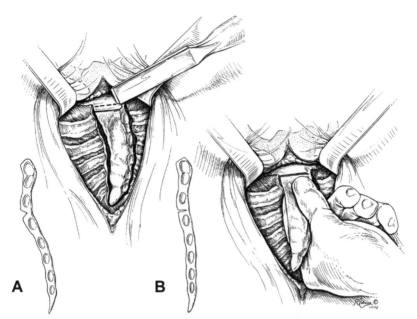

Fig. 16. The sternal bar is fixed to the lateral ribs and sternum. (*A*) The anterior sternal wedge is closed with 2 sutures. (*B*) The perichondrial sheaths are attached to the sternal edges. (*Reprinted from* Willekes CL, Backer CL, Mavroudis C. A 26-year review of pectus deformity repairs, including simultaneous intracardiac repair. Ann Thorac Surg 1999;67:513; with permission.)

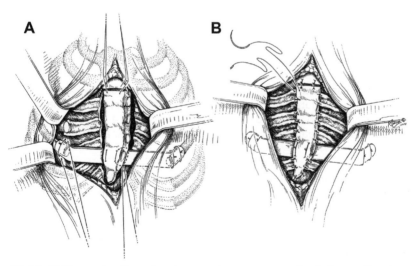

Fig. 17. (*A, B*) The pectoralis and rectus muscles are reapproximated over the sternum. Closed suction drains are placed above and below the muscle flaps. (*Reprinted from* Willekes CL, Backer CL, Mavroudis C. A 26-year review of pectus deformity repairs, including simultaneous intracardiac repair. Ann Thorac Surg 1999;67:514; with permission.)

drains (Hemovacs) are left beneath the pectoralis and skin flaps. The drains are removed when the output is 20 to 30 mL/d or less (usually postoperative day 3 or 4). A small chest tube or Blake drain is routinely placed in the right pleural space and removed on postoperative day 2. The sternal bar is removed through a small lateral incision as an outpatient procedure in the operating room 6 to 9 months post-operatively, except in children with Marfan syndrome, when it is removed 12 months later.

Results

Between 1972 and 2009, 198 children underwent repair of pectus deformity at the authors' institution. There were 175 pectus excavatum and 23 pectus carinatum and a 4:1 male predominance. One patient was referred for emergent open heart repair and pectus repair after attempted Nuss repair resulted in a perforated right atrium, perforated right ventricle, and partially disrupted tricuspid valve apparatus. Two patients were operated on after a failed Nuss operation. There were no deaths and only one significant complication, which required a return to the operating room for bleeding. In 1998, the authors reviewed long-term follow-up by means of a mailed questionnaire. Questionnaires were returned by 83% of patients and results were classified as excellent in 64 patients (64%), good in 25 (25%), fair in 8 (8%), and poor in 3 (3%). Patients in the current era for whom a sternal bar was used at the time of surgery reported excellent or good results 97% of the time. Similar results have been reported with repair of pectus carinatum.[47]

MINIMALLY INVASIVE REPAIR

Donald Nuss introduced a minimally invasive approach to pectus excavatum now known as the "Nuss operation," and published his 10-year results of the procedure in 1998.[48] Since that time it has gained widespread adoption among pediatric and thoracic surgeons. The technique is performed by placing 2 lateral incisions in the mid-axillary line at the level of the deepest convexity of the deformity. A thoracoscope is placed into the right pleural space through a separate incision. Bilateral thoracoscopy is used occasionally. An introducer is fed from one axillary incision to the other under thoracoscopic guidance. An umbilical tape is then pulled through to act as a guide for the individually curved Lorenz pectus bar, which is carefully pulled through facing up and then flipped down using the Lorenz rotational instrument. The pectus correction is assessed at this time and the curvature adjusted if necessary. The bar is fitted with bilateral stabilizing bars and secured to the chest wall with heavy suture. Patients are typically discharged from the hospital within 4 to 7 days. The bar is removed after 2 to 3 years as an outpatient procedure under anesthesia.

Results

Results of the minimally invasive repair of pectus excavatum from a large series were published by Hebra in 2000.[49] He reported good to excellent satisfaction rates in 93% of cases. There was a significant overall rate of complications of almost 20%, with the most common complication being reoperation for bar displacement. Additional complications included pneumothorax, pleural effusions, pericarditis, cardiac injury and, rarely, death.[50–52]

No large head-to-head studies of open repair versus minimally invasive repair have been published, although a nonrandomized clinical trial is currently underway.[53] The current procedure of choice remains the modified Ravitch repair, which the authors consider the "gold standard." This bias is based primarily on the superior safety with equivalent efficacy of the open repair compared with the minimally invasive procedure for a condition, which is relatively benign and has never been documented to affect longevity of life but merely lifestyle.[54,55] In its current form the authors do not believe this added risk is offset by the perceived benefit of smaller incisions.

REFERENCES

1. Oberhansli-Weiss I, Heymann MA, Rudolph AM, et al. The pattern and mechanisms of response to oxygen by the ductus arteriosus and umbilical artery. Pediatr Res 1972;6:693–700.
2. Clyman RI, Chan CY, Mauray F, et al. Permanent anatomic closure of the ductus arteriosus in newborn baboons: the roles of postnatal constriction, hypoxia, and gestation. Pediatr Res 1999;45:19–29.
3. Campbell M. Natural history of persistent ductus arteriosus. Br Heart J 1968;30: 4–13.
4. Mitchell SC, Korones SB, Berendes HW. Congenital heart disease in 56,109 births. Incidence and natural history. Circulation 1971;43:323–32.
5. Mitchell SC, Sellmann AH, Westphal MC, et al. Etiologic correlates in a study of congenital heart disease in 56,109 births. Am J Cardiol 1971;28:653–7.
6. Siassi B, Blanco C, Cabal LA, et al. Incidence and clinical features of patent ductus arteriosus in low-birth weight infants: a prospective analysis of 150 consecutively born infants. Pediatrics 1976;57:347–51.
7. Tutassaura H, Goldman B, Moes CA, et al. Spontaneous aneurysm of the ductus arteriosus in childhood. J Thorac Cardiovasc Surg 1969;57:180–4.
8. Stevenson JG, Kawabori I, Guntheroth WG. Pulsed Doppler echocardiographic diagnosis of patent ductus arteriosus: sensitivity, specificity, limitations, and technical features. Cathet Cardiovasc Diagn 1980;6:255–63.
9. Bridges ND, Mallory GB Jr, Huddleston CB, et al. Lung transplantation in children and young adults with cardiovascular disease. Ann Thorac Surg 1995;59:813–20.
10. Heymann MA, Rudolph AM, Silverman NH. Closure of the ductus arteriosus in premature infants by inhibition of prostaglandin synthesis. N Engl J Med 1976; 295:530–3.
11. Gersony WM, Peckham GJ, Ellison RC, et al. Effects of indomethacin in premature infants with patent ductus arteriosus: results of a national collaborative study. J Pediatr 1983;102:895–906.
12. Alexander F, Chiu L, Hammel J, et al. Analysis of outcome in 298 extremely low-birth-weight infants with patent ductus arteriosus. J Pediatr Surg 2009;44:112–7.
13. Cotton RB, Stahlman MT, Bender HW, et al. Randomized trial of early closure of symptomatic patent ductus arteriosus in small preterm infants. J Pediatr 1978;93: 647–51.
14. Pontius RG, Danielson GK, Noonan JA, et al. Illusions leading to surgical closure of the distal left pulmonary artery instead of the ductus arteriosus. J Thorac Cardiovasc Surg 1981;82:107.
15. Fleming WH, Sarafian LB, Kugler JD, et al. Ligation of patent ductus arteriosus in premature infants: importance of accurate anatomic definition. Pediatrics 1983; 71:373–5.
16. Potts WJ, Gibson S, Smith, et al. Diagnosis and surgical treatment of patent ductus arteriosus. Arch Surg 1949;58:612–22.
17. Gross RE. Complete division for the patent ductus arteriosus. J Thorac Surg 1947;16:314–22.

18. Musewe NN, Benson LN, Smallhorn JF, et al. Two-dimensional echocardiographic and color flow Doppler evaluation of ductal occlusion with the Rashkind prosthesis. Circulation 1989;80:1706–10.
19. Raaijmaakers B, Nijveld A, van Oort A, et al. Difficulties generated by the small, persistently patent, arterial duct. Cardiol Young 1999;9:392–5.
20. Gray DT, Fyler DC, Walker AM, et al. Clinical outcomes and costs of transcatheter as compared with surgical closure of patent ductus arteriosus. The Patent Ductus Arteriosus Closure Comparative Study Group. N Engl J Med 1993;329:1517–23.
21. Miles RH, DeLeon SY, Muraskas J, et al. Safety of patent ductus arteriosus closure in premature infants without tube thoracostomy. Ann Thorac Surg 1995; 59:668–70.
22. Mavroudis C, Backer CL, Gevitz M. Forty-six years of patent ductus arteriosus division at Children's Memorial Hospital of Chicago. Standards for comparison. Ann Surg 1994;220:402–9.
23. Omari BO, Shapiro S, Ginzton L, et al. Closure of short, wide patent ductus arteriosus with cardiopulmonary bypass and balloon occlusion. Ann Thorac Surg 1998;66:277–8.
24. Hines MH, Bensky AS, Hammon JW Jr, et al. Video-assisted thoracoscopic ligation of patent ductus arteriosus: safe and outpatient. Ann Thorac Surg 1998;66: 853–9.
25. Backer CL, Ilbawi MN, Idriss FS, et al. Vascular anomalies causing tracheoesophageal compression. Review of experience in children. J Thorac Cardiovasc Surg 1989;97:725–31.
26. Felson B, Palayew MJ. The two types of right aortic arch. Radiology 1963;81: 745–59.
27. Sade RM, Rosenthal A, Fellows K, et al. Pulmonary artery sling. J Thorac Cardiovasc Surg 1975;69:333–46.
28. Berdon WE, Baker DH, Wung JT, et al. Complete cartilage-ring tracheal stenosis associated with anomalous left pulmonary artery: the ring-sling complex. Radiology 1984;152:57–64.
29. Ardito JM, Ossoff RH, Tucker GF Jr, et al. Innominate artery compression of the trachea in infants with reflex apnea. Ann Otol Rhinol Laryngol 1980;89:401–5.
30. Backer CL, Mavroudis CM, Rigsby CK, et al. Trends in vascular ring surgery. J Thorac Cardiovasc Surg 2005;129:1339–47.
31. van Son JA, Julsrud PR, Hagler DJ, et al. Surgical treatment of vascular rings: the Mayo Clinic experience. Mayo Clin Proc 1993;68:1056–63.
32. McFaul R, Millard P, Nowicki E. Vascular rings necessitating right thoracotomy. J Thorac Cardiovasc Surg 1981;82:306.
33. Kommerell B. Verlagerung des osophagus durch eine abnorm verlaufende arteria subclavia dextra (arteria lusoria). Fortschr Geb Rontgenstr 1936;54:590–5 [in German].
34. Fisher RG, Whigham CJ, Trinh C. Diverticula of Kommerell and aberrant subclavian arteries complicated by aneurysms. Cardiovasc Intervent Radiol 2005;28: 553–60.
35. Backer CL, Hillman N, Mavroudis C, et al. Resection of Kommerell's diverticulum and left subclavian artery transfer for recurrent symptoms after vascular ring division. Eur J Cardio-thorac Surg 2002;22:64–9.
36. Moes CA, Izukawa T, Trusler GA. Innominate artery compression of the trachea. Arch Otolaryngol 1975;101:733–8.
37. Potts WJ, Holinger PH, Rosenblum AH. Anomalous left pulmonary artery causing obstruction to right main bronchus: report of a case. JAMA 1954;155:1409–11.

38. Backer CL, Idriss FS, Holinger LD, et al. Pulmonary artery sling. Results of surgical repair in infancy. J Thorac Cardiovasc Surg 1992;103:683–91.
39. Backer CL, Mavroudis C, Dunham ME, et al. Pulmonary artery sling: results with median sternotomy, cardiopulmonary bypass, and reimplantation. Ann Thorac Surg 1999;67:1738–45.
40. Tsang V, Murday A, Gillbe C, et al. Slide tracheoplasty for congenital funnel-shaped tracheal stenosis. Ann Thorac Surg 1989;48:632–5.
41. Grillo HC. Slide tracheoplasty for long-segment congenital tracheal stenosis. Ann Thorac Surg 1994;58:613–21.
42. Dayan SH, Dunham ME, Backer CL, et al. Slide tracheoplasty in the management of congenital tracheal stenosis. Ann Otol Rhinol Laryngol 1997;106:914–9.
43. Kocyildirim E, Kanani M, Roebuck D, et al. Long-segment tracheal stenosis: slide tracheoplasty and a multidisciplinary approach improve outcomes and reduce costs. J Thorac Cardiovasc Surg 2004;128:876–82.
44. Manning PB, Rutter MJ, Border WL. Slide tracheoplasty in infants and children: risk factors for prolonged postoperative ventilatory support. Ann Thorac Surg 2008;85:1187–92.
45. Haller JA Jr, Kramer SS, Lietman SA. Use of CT scans in selection of patients for pectus excavatum surgery: a preliminary report. J Pediatr Surg 1987;22:904–6.
46. Ravitch MM. The operative treatment of pectus excavatum. Ann Surg 1949;122:429–44.
47. Fonkalsrud E. Surgical correction of pectus carinatum: lessons learned from 260 patients. J Pediatr Surg 2008;43:1235–43.
48. Nuss D, Kelly RE Jr, Croitoru DP. 10-Year review of a minimally invasive technique for the correction of pectus excavatum. J Pediatr Surg 1998;33:545–52.
49. Hebra A, Swoveland B, Egbert M, et al. Outcome analysis of minimally invasive repair of pectus excavatum: review of 251 cases. J Pediatr Surg 2000;35:252–7.
50. Moss RL, Albanese CT, Reynolds M. Major complications after minimally invasive repair of pectus excavatum: case reports. J Pediatr Surg 2001;36:155.
51. Ueda K. A cardiac injury in the Nuss procedure for pectus excavatum. Jpn J Plast Surg 2007;50:437–42.
52. Castellani C, Schalamon J, Saxena AK, et al. Early complications of the Nuss procedure for pectus excavatum: a prospective study. Pediatr Surg Int 2008;24:659–66.
53. Kelly RE, Shamberger RC, Mellins RB, et al. Prospective multicenter study of surgical correction of pectus excavatum: design, perioperative complications, pain, and baseline pulmonary function facilitated by internet based data collection. J Am Coll Surg 2007;205:205–16.
54. Haller J, Scherer L, Turner C, et al. Evolving management of pectus excavatum based on a single institutional experience of 664 patients. Ann Thorac Surg 1989;209:578–82.
55. Wynn SR, Driscoll DJ, Ostrom NK, et al. Exercise cardiorespiratory function in adolescents with pectus excavatum. Observations before and after operation. J Thorac Cardiovasc Surg 1990;99:41–7.

Index

Note: Page numbers of article titles are in **boldface** type.

Surg Clin N Am 90 (2010) 1115–1123
doi:10.1016/S0039-6109(10)00118-0
0039-6109/10/$ – see front matter © 2010 Elsevier Inc. All rights reserved.

surgical.theclinics.com

United States Postal Service

Statement of Ownership, Management, and Circulation
(All Periodicals Publications Except Requestor Publications)

1. Publication Title	2. Publication Number	3. Filing Date
Surgical Clinics of North America	5 2 9 - 8 0 0 0	9/15/10

4. Issue Frequency	5. Number of Issues Published Annually	6. Annual Subscription Price
Feb, Apr, Jun, Aug, Oct, Dec	6	$291.00

7. Complete Mailing Address of Known Office of Publication (Not printer) (Street, city, county, state, and ZIP+4®)

Elsevier Inc.
360 Park Avenue South
New York, NY 10010-1710

Contact Person
Stephen Bushing

Telephone (Include area code)
215-239-3688

8. Complete Mailing Address of Headquarters or General Business Office of Publisher (Not printer)

Elsevier Inc., 360 Park Avenue South, New York, NY 10010-1710

9. Full Names and Complete Mailing Addresses of Publisher, Editor, and Managing Editor (Do not leave blank)

Publisher (Name and complete mailing address)

Kim Murphy, Elsevier, Inc., 1600 John F. Kennedy Blvd. Suite 1800, Philadelphia, PA 19103-2899

Editor (Name and complete mailing address)

Catherine Bewick, Elsevier, Inc., 1600 John F. Kennedy Blvd. Suite 1800, Philadelphia, PA 19103-2899

Managing Editor (Name and complete mailing address)

Catherine Bewick, Elsevier, Inc., 1600 John F. Kennedy Blvd. Suite 1800, Philadelphia, PA 19103-2899

10. Owner (Do not leave blank. If the publication is owned by a corporation, give the name and address of the corporation immediately followed by the names and addresses of all stockholders owning or holding 1 percent or more of the total amount of stock. If not owned by a corporation, give the names and addresses of the individual owners. If owned by a partnership or other unincorporated firm, give its name and address as well as those of each individual owner. If the publication is published by a nonprofit organization, give its name and address.)

Full Name	Complete Mailing Address
Wholly owned subsidiary of	4520 East-West Highway
Reed/Elsevier, US holdings	Bethesda, MD 20814

11. Known Bondholders, Mortgagees, and Other Security Holders Owning or Holding 1 Percent or More of Total Amount of Bonds, Mortgages, or Other Securities. If none, check box ☑ None

Full Name	Complete Mailing Address
N/A	

12. Tax Status (For completion by nonprofit organizations authorized to mail at nonprofit rates) (Check one)
The purpose, function, and nonprofit status of this organization and the exempt status for federal income tax purposes:
☐ Has Not Changed During Preceding 12 Months
☐ Has Changed During Preceding 12 Months (Publisher must submit explanation of change with this statement)

PS Form 3526, September 2007 (Page 1 of 3 (Instructions Page 3)) PSN 7530-01-000-9931 PRIVACY NOTICE: See our Privacy policy in www.usps.com

13. Publication Title	14. Issue Date for Circulation Data Below
Surgical Clinics of North America	August 2010

15. Extent and Nature of Circulation		Average No. Copies Each Issue During Preceding 12 Months	No. Copies of Single Issue Published Nearest to Filing Date
a. Total Number of Copies (Net press run)		3975	3800
b. Paid Circulation (By Mail and Outside the Mail)	(1) Mailed Outside-County Paid Subscriptions Stated on PS Form 3541. (Include paid distribution above nominal rate, advertiser's proof copies, and exchange copies)	1418	1405
	(2) Mailed In-County Paid Subscriptions Stated on PS Form 3541 (Include paid distribution above nominal rate, advertiser's proof copies, and exchange copies)		
	(3) Paid Distribution Outside the Mails Including Sales Through Dealers and Carriers, Street Vendors, Counter Sales, and Other Paid Distribution Outside USPS®	1400	1212
	(4) Paid Distribution by Other Classes Mailed Through the USPS (e.g. First-Class Mail®)		
c. Total Paid Distribution (Sum of 15b (1), (2), (3), and (4))	▲	2818	2617
d. Free or Nominal Rate Distribution (By Mail and Outside the Mail)	(1) Free or Nominal Rate Outside-County Copies Included on PS Form 3541	95	86
	(2) Free or Nominal Rate In-County Copies Included on PS Form 3541		
	(3) Free or Nominal Rate Copies Mailed at Other Classes Through the USPS (e.g. First-Class Mail)		
	(4) Free or Nominal Rate Distribution Outside the Mail (Carriers or other means)		
e. Total Free or Nominal Rate Distribution (Sum of 15d (1), (2), (3) and (4))	▲	95	86
f. Total Distribution (Sum of 15c and 15e)	▲	2913	2703
g. Copies not Distributed (See instructions to publishers #4 (page #3))	▲	1062	1097
h. Total (Sum of 15f and g)	▲	3975	3800
i. Percent Paid (15c divided by 15f times 100)		96.74%	96.82%

16. Publication of Statement of Ownership

☐ If the publication is a general publication, publication of this statement is required. Will be printed in the October 2010 issue of this publication. ☐ Publication not required

17. Signature and Title of Editor, Publisher, Business Manager, or Owner

Stephen R. Bushing — Fulfillment/Inventory Specialist

Stephen R. Bushing – Fulfillment/Inventory Specialist

Date
September 15, 2010

I certify that all information furnished on this form is true and complete. I understand that anyone who furnishes false or misleading information on this form or who omits material or information requested on the form may be subject to criminal sanctions (including fines and imprisonment) and/or civil sanctions (including civil penalties).

PS Form 3526, September 2007 (Page 2 of 3)

Moving?

Make sure your subscription moves with you!

To notify us of your new address, find your **Clinics Account Number** (located on your mailing label above your name), and contact customer service at:

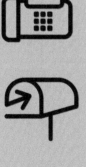

Email: journalscustomerservice-usa@elsevier.com

800-654-2452 (subscribers in the U.S. & Canada)
314-447-8871 (subscribers outside of the U.S. & Canada)

Fax number: 314-447-8029

Elsevier Health Sciences Division
Subscription Customer Service
3251 Riverport Lane
Maryland Heights, MO 63043

*To ensure uninterrupted delivery of your subscription, please notify us at least 4 weeks in advance of move.

Printed and bound by CPI Group (UK) Ltd, Croydon, CR0 4YY

03/10/2024

01040446-0003